THE
FEMININE
WARRIOR

A Woman's Guide
to Verbal,
Psychological,
and Physical
Empowerment

AL MARREWA

KENSINGTON BOOKS
http://www.kensingtonbooks.com

This book is available at quantity discounts with bulk purchase for educational, business, or promotional use. For information, please write: Special Sales Department, Kensington Publishing, 850 Third Avenue, New York, NY 10022.

KENSINGTON BOOKS are published by

Kensington Publishing Corp.
850 Third Avenue
New York, NY 10022

Copyright © 1998 by Al Marrewa
Drawings by Tommy Tejeda

Library of Congress Card Catalog Number: 97-073756
ISBN 1-57566-247-7

First Kensington Hardcover Printing: February, 1998
10 9 8 7 6 5 4 3 2 1

Printed in the United States of America

For my mother and father

ACKNOWLEDGMENTS

A heartfelt thank-you goes out to the following . . .

Denise Marcil, my agent
*You took a chance and you believed in me, and
for that I will be forever grateful.*

Marie Jansen Bayer, my "right hand"
*I couldn't have done it without you. Thank you for
your candor, intelligence, and untiring
commitment to this book.*

Tracy Bernstein, my editor
*My deepest appreciation for your guidance and
direction.*

Marianne Moloney, my mentor and friend
*Your words of wisdom and enthusiasm for this
project fueled my desire to make a difference.*

Jo Ann Haun
*Your editorial assistance was of great value and
much appreciated.*

Matthew Ember

*Your gift for teaching continues to feed my hunger
to become the best I can be, both on and off the
mat.*

Andre Salvage

*Thank you for opening the door and showing me
"the way." Your instruction has made an
everlasting impression upon my life.*

To all the women whom I have trained over the years . . .

*Your courage and strength have brought great
meaning to my life.*
*Thank you for helping me to grow as a man, and
as a human being.*

CONTENTS

x   **Contents**

xii Contents

Teaching is my purpose and my passion, and there is nothing in the world that I enjoy more. As a teacher and educator, I strive to motivate, guide, support, and challenge my students towards continual growth and enlightenment. I often say that the role of a teacher is to "open the door" for others. Naturally, the choice to walk through this door is up to each student, but truly great teachers make this choice the *only* choice for their students.

The door is now open. . . .

The daughter of a lion is also a lion.
—*Arabian proverb*

PREFACE

In 1986 I walked into a martial arts studio in Los Angeles, California, and my life changed forever. I couldn't have known it at the time, but my first day on the mat would eventually lead me into a new profession, and with it an approach to life that I might otherwise never have known.

In recent years, I have traveled across the country teaching personal empowerment to women of all ages. This experience has been a deeply rewarding one for me. I consider myself blessed to have met so many wonderful women through my work. With each and every program, I continue to gain new insights into the thoughts, feelings, perceptions, and concerns of women about such critical issues as violence, power, and gender roles.

If you're wondering how a man could write a book on the subject of female empowerment, or even understand it, the answer is, I didn't do it on my own. To a great extent, my expertise has been derived from the education *I* have received from my female students. I consider these women to be my co-authors because they proposed, shaped, and influenced so many of the ideas you will see presented in this book. In many ways, I see myself as a messenger for the life lessons experienced by these women. I pass these valuable lessons on to you, the reader, in the hope that they will empower you in every way imaginable.

Emotional, spiritual, psychological, and physical empowerment can all be yours. There's a marvelous link between one type of empowerment and another; each complements and strengthens the others. For example, I've found that women who excel at physical self-defense generally view themselves as empowered individuals at home, at work, and in their relationships. I've seen the transformation time and time again: self-defense training becomes an empowerment springboard for women who once felt powerless in many areas of their lives.

Kimberly* is a prime example of this. When she came to her first workshop, it was obvious that she brought with her some painful, debilitating life experiences. Kimberly's behavior, body language, and tone of voice communicated a general discomfort with herself and others.

I looked forward to working with Kimberly, confident that the all-day workshop would transform her as dramatically as it had transformed so many women before her. Sure enough, as the day progressed, she began to face her fears with great courage and strength. Our role-playing exercises allowed her to experiment with new verbal and physical skills. This was uncharted territory for Kimberly, as it is for the majority of my students. But Rome wasn't built in a day and construction had to start sometime. On that particular day, Kimberly began building herself a new life.

At the program's conclusion, Kimberly came up to me and gave me a warm hug. She thanked me for giving her a newly discovered sense of power. I assured her, however, it was nothing she hadn't already possessed. It was all there from the beginning; I'd simply helped her to discover it. I thanked *her* for giving me the opportunity to work with such a wonderful human being. Viewing her transformation from a timid and passive woman to a more empowered one had been a real joy. To this day, Kimberly credits her workshop experience with bringing her a sense of power and a control over her life which she had always dreamed of having.

The power to take control of your life lies within. Although some people feel more empowered than others, we all have the potential to achieve new heights of personal strength and confidence. Sometimes, like Kimberly, you just need a guide to point you in the right direction. As you read the following pages, think

---

*In the interests of privacy, all names have been changed.

of me as that guide and as a friend. Realize that my motivation for writing this book was a simple one: to share with you what others have shared with me. You can realize your full potential as a human being and discover more happiness, security, joy, and inner peace. I don't have all the answers, but I'm confident that whatever answers I do not have, you will.

Assault prevention provides the basis for many of the ideas, thoughts, insights, and lessons throughout this book. As you read on, however, never lose sight of the fact that true empowerment extends far beyond assault prevention and self-defense. Empowerment is a state of mind, an attitude, a way of life. It's also a process, a rite of passage, a journey towards self-fulfillment. So let the journey begin!

1
POWER TOOLS

Assertiveness: A Cornerstone of Personal Empowerment

The journey towards true empowerment is a gradual one, with many steps along the way. One of these steps is learning how to be assertive. While knowing how to be assertive will enhance your personal safety (if you can control a situation verbally, there's less likelihood that you'll need to control it physically), its benefits extend well beyond threatening situations. Assertiveness is something you will use every day of your life. It includes knowing how to stand up for yourself, how to influence others, and how to communicate effectively.

Assertiveness sounds so easy in principle. What could be simpler or more straightforward than telling some creep to "Get lost," or telling a store clerk, "I want my money back"? Yet being assertive is often easier said than done. One reason for this is the conditioning that many women receive from childhood. Even now, little girls are frequently encouraged to be compliant, easygoing, and nonconfrontational. This may make them more "likeable," more "easy to live with," but in terms of personal empowerment, it leaves them at a decided disadvantage.

A few years ago, I addressed a small group of women in downtown San Francisco. As I began to speak about assertiveness, a woman jumped up and said, "It's just not natural for a woman to be aggressive. That's a male trait, not a female one!" As often happens, my listener thought that assertiveness and aggressiveness were one and the same thing. In fact, the dictionary defines aggressiveness as "hostile" and assertiveness as "forceful and self-confident." There's a world of difference between them!

This difference can take time to understand. I've found that those students who live in urban areas (where confrontations with strangers are almost routine) find it easier to be aggressive. Yet they find it just as hard to be assertive as students from rural and suburban areas! Because they've come to see aggressiveness as a survival skill, it can be hard for these urban students to appreciate how much more appropriate and effective assertiveness can be at times. To illustrate what I mean, take the following scenario:

Two co-workers, a man and a woman, run into one another at the elevator. As the man good-naturedly compliments the woman on her recent promotion, he puts his arm around her shoulder. She welcomes the compliment, but not his arm around her shoulder.

If this woman says calmly yet firmly, "Listen, Bob, don't touch me like that," or "Take your arm off my shoulder," that's an assertive response. If she yells, "Get your damn hands off me!" (and I've seen it happen), that's an aggressive one.

If you feel your safety is threatened, an aggressive response *can* be the right way to go. But in most situations, you don't need to act hostile, nasty, or belligerent to hold your ground. Nor do you need to insult, degrade, or humiliate the other person. In certain situations, those kinds of behaviors can be provocative and even dangerous. Assertiveness, on the other hand, should be a fixture of your daily life.

Sending a strong message is lesson one. Many women weaken an otherwise assertive response by phrasing it the wrong way. They usually do so without realizing it: they *think* they're delivering an assertive response, but they really aren't. They may phrase their message politely; for example:

"Please leave me alone."
"I wish you would go away."
"Excuse me, but that's none of your business."
"I would appreciate it if you'd stop that."

Or, they may phrase their message in the form of a question. Here are a few examples which I *do not* recommend:

"Would you mind cutting that out?"
"Would you just go away?"
"Do you think that's appropriate behavior?"
"What do you think you're doing?"

Finally, many women make the mistake of apologizing for their feelings:

"You're standing too close to me. *I'm sorry,* but it's making me feel uncomfortable."
"I'm sorry, but I'm just not interested."
"I'm sorry, but I want you to leave."

Or perhaps they make all these mistakes at once: "I'm sorry, but would you please leave me alone?"

In addition, some women feel they have to justify or explain their feelings at length. They get into a dialogue with their aggressor or harasser. Don't fall into the same trap. Assertive messages are short, direct, and to the point; that's what gives them impact. They don't invite discussion.

Assertiveness is the real bridge between verbal and physical empowerment. Quite frankly, if you find assertiveness difficult, you'll find nearly every other empowerment technique impossible. If you find it difficult to be direct in confrontational situations, think for a moment about situations where you do feel in control. If you're a parent, for example, chances are you already know how to be assertive with your child. And you know instinctively that the more direct your instructions are, the better: "Don't play with matches," for example, or "Look both ways before crossing the street." Not only your words but your body language, facial expression, and tone of voice make it clear that you mean business.

And believe me, what works with children can and will work with adults.

If you want to deliver a truly assertive message, follow these simple rules:

1. Be direct.
2. Never precede a statement with "please," "I wish," "excuse me," "I would appreciate," or any other words or phrases that weaken your message.
3. Never phrase your message in the form of a question. When you ask the other person to do something, you hand over your power. You imply that he has a choice.
4. Never apologize for the way you feel.

Apologizing can be a hard habit to break. Whenever students try a fighting technique on me, they usually apologize afterwards. If they yell at me during a role-playing exercise, they worry about hurting my feelings. And if I demonstrate a technique on my assistant, they invariably feel sorry for him. I have to assure them that he's highly paid and heavily padded. More importantly, I urge them to get rid of their apologetic attitudes altogether; they have no place in the empowerment equation.

The Diplomatic Approach

There's more than one way to be assertive. With a stranger on the street, you can be brutally direct (more about that later). There will be times, however, when you'll need to be assertive with people you already know: friends, relatives, co-workers, neighbors, even your husband or boyfriend. On these occasions, I recommend that you couple your "commands" with something positive:

"I had a wonderful time tonight, but now it's time for you to leave."
"I enjoy working with you, but I find your jokes offensive."
"You're my husband *and I love you,* but don't talk to me that way."

Clearly, this is a gentler approach than one you'd use with a stranger. But in case you think it weakens your message, notice that each of these examples ends with a definite statement. They don't invite discussion. Your aim is not to tell the other person off or put him in his place, but to calmly and firmly communicate what you want.

Most of us find it easier to be assertive with strangers than with people we know. The closer the relationship, the more we worry about causing offense or hurting someone's feelings. However, I can't overemphasize how important it is to be assertive with acquaintances, friends, and relatives. Many of the women who attend my seminars have been victims of rape or assault and *nearly 80 percent of them* were attacked by someone they knew. An aggressor may spend weeks, months, even years testing a woman's boundaries. If she doesn't respond assertively, the testing will just continue. Her aggressor will become bolder and may be encouraged to initiate an actual physical assault.

If someone has been bothering you, harassing you, or crossing one of your physical boundaries, it's never too late to put a stop to it.

Practice Makes Perfect

Assertiveness is not something that any of us learn overnight, and let's face it, some people are just naturally more assertive than others. Unfortunately, if you have trouble standing up to shop clerks (for example), it's no use thinking you'll be assertive in a threatening situation.

To improve your assertiveness skills you need to practice them every day. The best thing to do is start "small," then gradually work up from there; we all need to crawl before we can walk. For example, you might begin by asking shop clerks for more prompt assistance. Then, as you gain more confidence in your assertiveness skills, work up to asking your boss for a raise. And keep in mind that assertiveness needn't always be confrontational. It can also be positive, as when you thank a waitress for giving you good service. Either way, try to express yourself! Say what's on your mind. Every time you do this it will become a little easier. Improvement is guaranteed!

An assertive woman respects the rights and feelings of others, yet she's also willing to risk their rejection or disapproval. She knows that being true to herself is more important than pleasing others. She realizes that "people-pleasers" are not empowered individuals.

I used to be a real people-pleaser, reluctant to stand up for myself in many situations for fear of causing offense. Ironically, this didn't change even after I began to learn the martial arts. There I was, studying for a black belt, but if a waiter brought me the wrong dinner, I'd eat it anyway!

That started to change when I sat in on a women's self-defense class. Hearing the instructor emphasize the importance of assertiveness, I began to understand that it complements physical self-defense, and vice versa. One supports the other. Once I learned how to be assertive in my daily life, I found that it enhanced my fighting skills to an unbelievable degree. More importantly, I was on the road from being a good martial artist to becoming an empowered human being.

I remember getting a call from Debbie. She wanted me to know that just hours after completing her empowerment training, she had put it into practice. Hearing the excitement and pride in Debbie's voice, I half expected to hear that she'd deterred a physical assault. In fact, her experience was rather different. For many weeks, a friend had been asking to borrow a rather expensive camera. Debbie didn't want to loan her the camera, so she kept stalling or trying to duck the woman's calls. When they did speak, she said things like, "I'm not sure," or "Let me think about it." However, once she learned that she could be assertive without being aggressive or insulting, Debbie was able to call the woman up and say, "You're a dear friend, but I don't want to loan you my camera. It's just not something I feel comfortable doing."

To some people, that simple act of assertiveness might seem like nothing. But for Debbie it was a personal milestone, a turning point. The first step is always the hardest, and she had taken her first small but significant step in the right direction. And so often, the road to personal empowerment is paved with little victories like hers.

Evelyn faced a difficult situation at work. One of the vendors who came to her office kept asking her out. She politely told him she just wasn't interested, but he still wouldn't leave her alone. On two occasions, he actually stopped her from closing the door to her office. The relationship with that vendor was valuable to her company, so it was hard for Evelyn to see a way out of her dilemma.

After completing her assertiveness training, Evelyn decided to do three things which she hadn't done before. First, she would tell the vendor "no" forcefully and emphatically, supporting her words with appropriate body language. Second, she would tell others in her department and throughout the company what was happening; this would bring her problem out of the closet. Third, she would ensure that someone else was with her when she met with this vendor in the future.

As it turned out, Evelyn didn't need to take the second and third steps. Once she told him that there was no way she would ever go out with him, the vendor finally got the message. He never harassed her again.

Is there someone in your own life who by word or deed makes you feel uncomfortable? It could be anyone: a co-worker, an acquaintance, even a close friend or family member. One student with two young children had an older sister who persisted in using profanity around them; another had a brother-in-law who was a bit too familiar with his hugs and kisses. Initially, another woman couldn't think of anyone who was crossing her personal boundaries. But after Maggie and I talked more about it, she remembered that her aunt was always grilling her about the state of her marriage, asking intrusive questions that made Maggie feel very uncomfortable. Once she realized this, Maggie was able to confront her aunt and say, "You know I love you, but I want you to stop asking me about my marriage." Simple as that. She stuck to her guns until her aunt eventually got the point.

Is there someone who harasses you, or touches you in an inappropriate way? Does his or her conduct intimidate, bother, or just plain frighten you? Your safety may not necessarily be in question; there may be someone who throws sexist comments, offensive jokes, or unwelcome questions your way. Either way, I urge you to confront that person as soon as possible.

I have no doubt that you'll find plenty of opportunities to practice your assertiveness skills. While there's a good chance you will never face a life-threatening situation, I have yet to meet a woman who hasn't been harassed, threatened, or just plain intimidated. As we all know, there's more than one way to be pushed around.

The Femininity Factor

Many women shrink from being assertive because they feel it's unfeminine. Don't believe it for a minute! Assertiveness and femininity can and should go together.

I've always been impressed by how even the most timid woman becomes a "feminine warrior" when one of her children is threatened. One reason she finds it easier to be assertive in this situation is that she knows public opinion is on her side: society approves of the woman who forcefully protects her children. But if she uses that same assertiveness to protect *herself,* there are still people who will label her unwomanly. Don't pay any attention to outdated definitions of femininity! Stand up for yourself with the same assertiveness that you would use to protect your child.

The "Helpless Female"

Many women retreat into the role of the "helpless female" when confronted with an unpleasant situation. It's important to recognize that this is yet another conditioned response, encouraged since childhood. It's a relic from Victorian times, when society viewed helplessness as an attractively feminine characteristic.

Ask yourself if you're likely to fall into the same role. If you were at a party and a man spoke to you in an offensive way, what would you do? Would you confront him yourself, or ask your husband or boyfriend to set him straight? If a co-worker touched you in a manner you found inappropriate, would you tell him off, or head to the personnel department to file a sexual harassment complaint? If you were on the street and thought a man was following you, would you confront him? Or would your first thought be to find a police officer or male protector?

There are times when asking another person for help *is* a good idea. But whenever possible, try to resolve the situation yourself. By doing so, you retain and exercise your power. You'll also find that standing up for yourself is wonderfully self-supporting: the more you do it, the easier it gets.

Be Ready For A Reaction

A man or woman says something inappropriate to you for one of two reasons: because they didn't realize it would make you feel uncomfortable, or because they did. Either way, your response should be the same. The beauty of an assertive response (as opposed to a meek or aggressive one) is that it works in either situation.

Whenever you respond assertively, however, be prepared for a reaction. Obviously, you'd welcome an apology: "I'm sorry, I didn't realize that bothered you." That's certainly the ideal response, but apologies are usually the exception to the rule. The other person is far more likely to become defensive or hostile. Here are a few examples of a defensive response:

"You're getting the wrong idea."
"I didn't mean anything by that!"
"I was just being friendly."
"Hey, I'm not that kind of guy."

And here are some hostile ones:

"You're just too sensitive."
"Don't tell me what to do!"
"What's your problem?!"

Notice that most of these statements invite a response. Don't rise to the bait! Say "I don't want to hear about it" or "End of discussion," then walk away.

Intuition: Your Inner Voice

Intuition is that feeling you've had at one time or another that "something wasn't right" or that something was about to happen. Until I started teaching personal empowerment, I never gave much thought to intuition. Like most people, I'd been encouraged since childhood to value rational, analytical thinking over hunches and gut feelings. But as I began meeting women who had survived rape and assault, I discovered that many if not all of them shared a similar experience: they'd all had a sense of foreboding before they were attacked. Their intuition, or "inner voice," had warned them of impending danger.

Many sexual harassers and attackers give off subtle clues to their intentions. Listening to your intuition will help you recognize those clues. One of my students recalled feeling uneasy when a co-worker brushed up against her one day at the office. She chose to push her feelings aside, however, reasoning that because she knew him she could trust him. Sadly, she was raped by this man just two weeks later.

On the positive side, another student remembers an occasion when she *did* listen to her intuition. Suzanne was at a fairly raucous party, and late into the evening began to feel uncomfortable. So she took a moment to figure out *why*. That's when she realized that the other women had left the party, and the remaining men were well past their first drinks. Before she'd even stopped to think about it, Suzanne's inner voice had warned her, *It's time for you to leave.*

Listen to your intuition. It's real, not imagined. Your inner voice always speaks the truth, so never doubt it, ignore it, or suppress it. When your intuition sets off warning bells, change the situation immediately and get to a safe place.

The benefits of intuition go well beyond personal safety: it will also help you in your daily life. There was once a time when I was programmed to leave my intuition by the side of the road, unaware that without this essential "power tool" I probably had a less than fifty-fifty chance of making the right choice in any situation. Looking back, I now realize that much of the pain I experienced in personal relationships stemmed from my total disregard for my intuition. When I walked down the aisle on my wedding day, for example, I knew full well that I was making a mistake; my inner voice was speaking the truth. But like so many people do, I chose to ignore that voice. If only I had listened to my intuition, I might have avoided the pain of a failed marriage that ended in divorce. As it was, I learned a valuable lesson: one's intuition should never be denied.

Intuition is a valuable tool in making decisions of any kind. The head should always be coupled with the heart. In other words, come to a preliminary decision through rational, level-headed thinking, then confirm that decision by consulting your inner voice. Ultimately, your intuition should have the final say.

To get in touch with your intuition, use this simple, four-step approach:

1. Find a quiet place.
2. Be still.
3. Listen to your inner voice.
4. Follow what you hear.

Once you appreciate the power of intuition, making the right decisions will become so much easier. While you'll continue to weigh the pros and cons of every option, at the end of this rational, intellectual process, you'll consult your inner voice. In questionable, confusing, or dangerous situations, your intuition is a guiding light that will always lead you down the right path.

Body Language: The Silent Communicator

Body language is more powerful than the spoken word. It includes your walk, your posture, eye contact, facial expression, and overall appearance. How you feel about yourself and your surroundings is reflected in how you carry yourself. Your body language will tell others if you're strong and secure, or anxious and uncertain.

I recall reading about a woman who was raped in the parking lot of a popular Los Angeles department store. Thankfully, she survived the attack and her assailant was arrested soon afterward. The interesting thing about this case was the rapist's confession to the police. As he explained, he liked to sit in his car in the parking lot and watch shoppers exit the store. He would spend hours, even days, sizing up potential victims, and not until he'd spotted the right target would he make his move.

Contrary to popular belief, this rapist wasn't looking for the most attractive woman or the one in the shortest skirt: he was looking for signs of weakness. Women who were aware of their surroundings and confident in their demeanor were not good candidates; they spelled trouble. He preferred individuals who seemed unsure of themselves or their surroundings. These women were easy to spot, he bragged: their body language said it all. He especially favored women who appeared confused or lost as they searched the lot for their cars; these he considered to be prime targets. As you can see, body language is vital to communication even when you can't see who you're communicating with.

Even though you may be feeling anxious in a particular situation, you can use your body language to give just the opposite impression. Body language is sometimes a form of acting; you can use it to "play the role" of a fearless and self-assured person. This does more than discourage potential attackers, I might add. The more you pretend to be confident, the more confident you'll actually start to feel. Stay alert, hold your head high, keep your back straight and your stride deliberate. Those who communicate confidence and self-respect with their bodies are less likely to become victims of violent crime. Harassers and attackers tend to avoid this kind of person.

Your body language can also help you in everyday life, such as during a job interview or a stressful confrontation. In any situation where you want to appear confident, assertive, and in control, here are some examples of the right and wrong body language to use:

Right	*Wrong*
Sitting well back in your chair	Perching on the edge of your chair
Sitting up straight	Leaning forward

Facing the other person	Turning your body away
Keeping "solid" and still	Fidgeting; shifting from foot to foot
Making direct eye contact	Looking down or away
Keeping a calm expression	Rapid blinking; pursing or biting your lips
Keeping your hands relaxed	Playing with your hair or jewelry
Giving a firm handshake	Giving a weak handshake
Speaking up	Mumbling; speaking too softly
Taking your time to speak	Speaking too fast; interrupting
Filling your "personal space"	Trying to look "smaller" (slouching, rounding your shoulders, crossing your arms, etc.)

When you're feeling confident, confident body language just comes naturally. It's in situations where you're nervous, uncertain, or afraid that it becomes an effort, a real act of will. Nevertheless, assertive body language can be a triumph of perception over reality: while feeling nervous and afraid on the inside you focus on what you're communicating on the outside.

Assertive body language—and the lack of it—also plays a role in that proverbial minefield of male and female relationships. Even today, I still hear men insisting that, "When a girl says no she really means yes." This myth stubbornly refuses to die, and I think it has its roots in the fact that all of us, at one time or another, have said one thing while our body language communicated another.

Ambiguity is the enemy of clear communication. Let's say, for example, that a man is pressuring you for a date. You tell him you're not interested. As you do so, however, you look away, or down at the ground. You avoid his eyes. You shift from one foot to another. So while you may be saying "no," your body language is communicating "I don't know," "Maybe," or "I'm not sure." Talk about mixed messages!

Anytime you communicate verbally, pay attention to your body language. Make sure it supports and underlines your words. Body language and assertiveness go hand in hand, and in a later segment ("Moving in the Right Direction"), I'll teach you more about using body language to strengthen your message.

* * *

Assertiveness, intuition, and body language will bring you a degree of personal empowerment you may never have known before. Best of all, you can start practicing these skills *today*. Continue to use them on a daily basis, and you'll experience the confidence and sense of power that they invariably provide.

2
LIVING SMART

An Ounce of Prevention

When I address an audience on the subject of personal safety, I can almost hear a collective yawn. Let's face it: in the arena of self-empowerment, safety measures will never be as dramatic or interesting as assertiveness or a knee to the groin. The fact remains, however, that you cannot be empowered unless you are safe, and the very best way to protect yourself from dangerous situations is to avoid them altogether. This approach may strike you as passive, defensive, even downright boring. But believe me, it's always the smartest way to go.

We're all vulnerable to the cruel realities of crime. And before you do anything to protect yourself, you must acknowledge this vulnerability. If I've learned nothing else through my work teaching personal empowerment, it's that anyone can be a victim of harassment or violence, regardless of their sex, age, race, religion, occupation, or level of physical fitness. You've heard this before; you probably accept it in principle. But do you really accept it in practice? Most people live in a state of denial. It's part of human nature to feel that it will not, could not, "happen to me."

In Tom Wolfe's *The Right Stuff*, he described a group of professional test pilots who denied their own vulnerability even as their comrades were dying in crashes left and right. Clinging to logical reasons for each fatality ("He waited too long to lower his flaps," "He forgot to check his oxygen system," etc.), they refused to acknowledge that the same thing could happen to them. We do the very same thing when we hear about violent crime, looking for reasons why it could not happen to us. A prostitute is murdered? *She was in a dangerous line of work.* A tourist is mugged on the subway? *He should have known the subway was dangerous.* A co-worker is raped? *She was walking alone after dark.* You get the idea. Yet the reality is that you may live and work in a "good" area, take every sensible precaution, and still fall victim to violent crime. I had one student who recognized her vulnerability—and acted accordingly—while traveling through high-crime areas, only to be carjacked while parked in Beverly Hills.

I'm not encouraging you to live in fear, to feel so vulnerable to crime that you're inhibited from trying new things or taking certain risks. What I do want you to do is keep your eyes wide open, to live in a state of awareness rather than denial. Acknowledging your vulnerability gives you an edge, helping you to avoid not just violent crime, but harassment and victimization in all their many forms.

It's ironic, but I've found that martial arts training has made me *more* aware of my own vulnerability. I hold a sixth degree black belt, but not for a moment do I believe that this makes me invulnerable to violent crime. Quite the opposite, in fact: compared to the average Joe, I have a healthier respect for the risks of the street. Yet rather than feeling crippled by this awareness, I feel empowered by it.

Sir Francis Bacon said it best: "Knowledge itself is power." And acknowledging your vulnerability empowers you to take the next important step: take responsibility for your own safety.

When Harry Truman became president, he put a sign on his desk that read "The buck stops here." And when it comes to your personal safety, the buck always stops with you. Unfortunately, taking responsibility for anything has become a rare commodity in recent years. Just look at the explosion of personal injury lawsuits, the "hot coffee" suit against McDonald's being a notorious example. And more and more, governments, politicians, corporations, and criminal defendants are taking the easy way out and passing the buck of responsibility.

This mind-set becomes downright dangerous when it comes to personal safety. I'm always amazed at the number of people who dismiss the whole idea of self-defense, insisting "I just don't want to think about it," or "There's nothing I can do." Both viewpoints abdicate personal responsibility. So, too, does a reliance on other people. Depending on others for your protection leads to a false sense of security which increases your chances of being victimized.

The single biggest mistake women make in this regard is depending on men for protection. Abby's story illustrates this perfectly:

> I'd always prided myself on my ability to look after myself. I'd lived in Chicago my whole life, so I was pretty streetwise. I didn't take chances. When I drove into the garage under my building, I always took a good look around before I got out of my car. I took the elevator, never the stairs. I had my house keys ready so I wouldn't have to stop and search for them. You might say I did everything right.
>
> One night after a party, I arrived home with my boyfriend. Greg is a six foot tall bodybuilder who played football in college: just the kind of guy people do not mess with. I always felt safer with him, and that's probably why, on that particular night, I broke all my own rules.
>
> Greg got impatient waiting for the elevator and headed for the stairs. I remember feeling a twinge of uncertainty, but I ignored it. As I followed him up the stairs, a man suddenly came out of nowhere. Greg was shoved backwards down the stairs; he broke two ribs in the fall and suffered a mild concussion. Waving a knife, the attacker shoved me against the wall. Then he grabbed my purse and took off.
>
> I count myself lucky that I wasn't badly hurt. If that mugger had been a rapist, Greg wouldn't have been able to help me; he was really down for the count. I can tell you this: never again will I depend on someone else for my protection.

Contrary to popular belief, most men know absolutely nothing about self-defense. Too often, they assume that the power of a "good left hook" or their sheer advantage in size and strength will carry them through. Unfortunately, the street is neither a boxing ring nor a football field, and a man's size and strength count for little when it comes to vicious assault. And anyone, man or woman, can be taken by surprise.

Even when they're smart enough to doubt their own abilities, most men would rather die than tell you, "I'm sorry, but I'm not sure I can protect you." The macho ethic is just too strong; our role as protectors of women has been instilled in many of us since childhood. So when it comes to personal safety, remember: the only person you should ever rely upon is (you guessed it!) you.

Depending on others for our safety is akin to depending on doctors for our physical well-being. Certainly, doctors are there if things go wrong; they may even practice preventive medicine. Yet you must still eat right, exercise, and so on because you know that safeguarding your health is ultimately your responsibility. Likewise, because budget and manpower restrictions don't allow the police to focus on crime prevention, we've had to assume some responsibility for our own safety by installing alarm systems or forming neighborhood watch groups. Whenever possible, extend this self-reliant attitude into your daily life. Remember that other people are nothing more than backup: while they may enhance your safety, they can't ensure it.

Safety as a Way of Life

As you already know, the best way to protect yourself from fires is to take preventive measures such as installing smoke alarms and keeping matches away from children. It's no different with self-defense. Although self-defense techniques are invaluable in certain situations, the very best way to protect yourself from assault is to adopt a whole new way of life.

To begin with, make your safety your top priority. That may sound obvious, but most people don't do it. When I ask new students to list their priorities, they routinely cite family, career, home, job, and so on. Not one has included personal safety on her list. But, truth is, nothing else matters if you aren't safe.

We all have different priorities, so take the time to examine yours. Let's say, for example, that you like to exercise. Burning calories is important to you, so you jog. Your time schedule is tight, so you have to run at dusk. Solitude is important to you, so you run alone. Once you make safety your *top* priority, however, you might opt to run earlier in the day, run with a friend, or work out in a gym instead.

Maybe your job is very important to you. So you stay late at the office, even if that means working alone in the building, or walking through a deserted garage to reach your car. Once safety is your top priority, however, you might put in those extra hours in the morning, or find a co-worker to accompany you to your car after dark. With every decision that you make, always consider the safety factor.

If you approach personal safety as a *lifestyle,* setting priorities will become second nature. You'll begin to assess your safety level automatically, regardless of where you are or whom you're with.

Now let's talk about planning. Because most assaults are planned, *you* must plan in order to stay one step ahead of a potential attacker. Unfortunately, most people don't start planning until they're actually in danger: when they find themselves in a deserted parking lot, for example, or isolated in an elevator with a stranger. By then it may be too late. The best time to plan is *now,* while you're safe. Don't wait until your safety is in question: that's like preparing for an earthquake after the ground begins to shake!

In later chapters, I'll give you specific tips on how, when, and where to plan for your safety. For now, I want you to understand the importance of mental planning. The value of thinking ahead can't be underestimated, and developing a heightened sense of awareness will help you plan. The more aware you are, the more likely you are to spot possible dangers in advance.

Because most of us lead hectic lives, we're usually too busy to concentrate on our surroundings. Unfortunately, when your thoughts are racing in a hundred different directions, personal safety invariably takes a back seat, and it's precisely when your mind is elsewhere that you're most at risk.

As busy as we may get, however, we still remain aware of certain things. Take traffic, for example: we know we have to look both ways before crossing a busy street. Now try to extend this awareness to include the *people* around you. Wherever you are— at work, at school, out in public, or even out with friends—

remember: your eyes and ears are your very best defense. If you're walking down the sidewalk, take note of your surroundings. Maybe two teenagers are loitering in a doorway; up ahead, there's another guy asking for change. Ask yourself, "Are any of them likely to give me trouble? Should I turn back? Cross to the other side of the street? Hail a cab?" Do this whether you're alone or with a companion.

Many women stay alert when out in public alone, but drop their guard as soon as they're with a man. With that male "protector" at their side, they don't feel they have to pay as much attention to potential dangers ("That's *his* job!"). But this idea that men can protect women *just because they are men* has to be one of the most insidious, debilitating myths that women are conditioned to believe. It does nothing but encourage women to be dependent, weak, and disempowered, so set it aside as you would any other myth. When it comes to personal safety, there's no substitute for doing the job yourself.

Trust as the Weapon of Choice

Whenever I conduct a seminar, I invite the audience to participate in a visualization exercise. I ask everyone to close their eyes and "visualize an attacker": not just the color of his hair, eyes, and skin, but his height, weight, dress, and demeanor. I ask them to study his face in great detail. Again and again, I say: "Picture this guy as if he's standing right in front of you."

Finally, I tell everyone to open their eyes. Then I ask them, "Did any of you visualize *me* during that exercise?" Not surprisingly, the answer to my question is always no. No one in the audience saw me as a potential attacker because they all trusted me. Bad move! Trust is the weapon of choice when it comes to many violent crimes, especially rape. If an attacker can gain your trust, you're in trouble.

One reason why my audience trusted me was because of how I looked. With my nice suit and tie, polished shoes, clean shave, and fresh haircut, I didn't fit the image of a dangerous person. It's a common mistake. We routinely trust people based on their appearance. The case of serial killer Ted Bundy is a perfect example: his victims willingly handed over their trust because he just didn't "look" like a killer. But the truth is that a rapist or killer can look like anyone.

Years ago, I was in a drugstore waiting to have a prescription filled. A young woman was in line ahead of me. As she stepped up to the counter, she gave the pharmacist personal information (name, address, telephone number) that I couldn't help but overhear. This was information that I easily could have used against her had I been a rapist. This woman had seen me standing right behind her. But having pegged me as a nicely dressed businessman, perhaps, she probably assumed that I was "safe," not realizing that you can never assume anything when it comes to personal safety. She foolishly handed over her trust to me, a trust I had not earned. Ideally, she would have written down the information being requested and therefore kept it confidential.

If we trust people based on their appearance, we also do so based on their profession, their status as authority figures, or simply because they've assured us, "Don't worry, you can trust me." Or we accept other people's assessments: trusting a date we know nothing about, for example, because someone *else* said he was a great guy. Society encourages all of us (but women in particular) to adopt this attitude, to give others the benefit of the doubt.

In Los Angeles in November 1995, the local news reported on the disappearance of model Linda Sobek, a former cheerleader for the Los Angeles Raiders football team. She was last known to have gone on a photo shoot with an unknown photographer. In cooperation with law enforcement, friends and family conducted an aggressive search for Sobek, distributing fliers with her picture and physical description. Concerns for her safety grew with each passing day.

Around the same time, I conducted a seminar for a local investment firm. At its conclusion, I handed out confidential evaluation forms to each of the participants. A week later, one of these forms came back from a woman named Maria, who wrote: "A member of our church was abducted and she is now missing. The women in our group need to know how to protect themselves and become aware that it can happen to even *good* women." When I saw the name of the church, I knew right away who Maria was referring to: Linda Sobek. The pastor from their church had been interviewed on the evening news the night before. And a few days later, with the assistance of the prime suspect, police were led to the Angeles National Forest; there, Sobek's body had been buried in a shallow grave.

Since that time, the photographer who hired Sobek has been tried and convicted of her murder. Clearly, she was killed by someone she thought that she could trust.

You might say that Linda Sobek fit the description of a "nice" woman: she worked hard, she had friends and family, she went to church. Neither by temperament or lifestyle did she go looking for trouble. The sad reality is, however, that anyone can be a victim of violent crime. I saw her case as a warning, an example of why trust should never be handed over lightly. I couldn't help but think that if I had spoken at her church—and been able to give that warning to Linda Sobek—her tragedy just might have been avoided. I was able to reach Maria, but not Linda, and that fact bothers me to this day.

Trust and The Good Samaritan

Good people help those in need, bad people don't: right? The answer is, *not always*. Many attackers, especially rapists, play the role of the Good Samaritan to win a woman's trust and lure her into their trap.

The Good Samaritan targets the woman who appears to need help. He just happens to be there when she locks herself out of her apartment, or when she's loaded down with groceries. He uses friendliness, kindness, and sincerity to gain her trust, then uses that trust against her.

> *When Sheri's car broke down on the highway, a man stopped to offer her a lift. She was tempted by the offer; the nearest phone was several miles away. And because he seemed so nice, so chivalrous, she didn't want to appear rude or ungrateful for his help. So she accepted the lift. Her Good Samaritan drove her to a more isolated spot, dragged her from the car, and raped her.*

Ideally, Sheri would have rebuffed that man's offer altogether, telling him calmly and firmly, "Thanks, but help is on the way." That wouldn't have left her stranded, by the way: as I'll explain in a later section, women do have other options in this kind of situation. Just keep in mind that accepting a lift—and blindly trusting a stranger—should never be one of them.

Before I knew about the Good Samaritan and his modus operandi, I'd go out of my way to help a woman in need; it seemed the gentlemanly thing to do. Seldom, if ever, did a woman turn my assistance down. Whether they were prompted by politeness, guilt, or true need, most accepted my aid without question. One woman actually allowed me to drag a piece of furniture into her apartment. If I'd been a rapist or attacker, she would have given me just the opening I needed. In retrospect, I realize that my behavior was not only sexist (I wouldn't help a man with *his* groceries), but misguided. It encouraged those women to accept help from others in the future. It reinforced their false sense of security.

In a switch on the Good Samaritan concept, an attacker may also pretend to need *your* help, exploiting your kindness and sympathy in order to win your trust. For example, he may pretend that his car has broken down ("Could you give me a lift to a gas station?"), or has locked himself out of his apartment ("Could I use your phone to call my landlord?"). Ted Bundy used this ruse to deadly effect. With his arm in a sling and a phony cast (in order to look disabled), he would ask his victim to help him move something heavy or load it into his trunk. Then as soon as she dropped her guard, he would attack.

When you appear self-sufficient, confident, and in control, you decrease your chances of being approached by a Good Samaritan. And keep in mind: the pitfalls of blindly handing over your trust extend well beyond assault situations. Before you trust anyone— a doctor, salesman, taxi driver, repairman, you name it—ask yourself, "What do I know about this person? What has he or she done to earn my trust?"

Am I saying to you, "Never trust anyone"? Absolutely not. But the trust you place in others should always be earned. Never give it without good reason; once you do, you place your welfare in their hands.

Trust and power go hand in hand. When you give someone your trust, you give them power. Although there are times when your safety is beyond your control, anything you can control, you should control. Stack the cards in your favor whenever possible, and your safety will be greatly enhanced.

Holding Your Ground: Setting and Protecting Your Boundaries

Simply put, your boundaries are those lines that, when crossed, make you feel uncomfortable. If you've ever felt that someone was intruding into your "space," then a boundary was being crossed. That person may have violated one of your *physical* boundaries (standing too close, or touching you in a manner you felt was inappropriate) or one of your *invisible* boundaries (asking intrusive questions, using offensive language, etc.).

Would you allow someone to cross your threshold and enter your home unless you'd invited him in? Of course not. The same should hold true for all your other boundaries. No one should talk to you in a familiar way, invade your personal space, or lay a hand on you unless you want him to. Boundary-setting has benefits that extend well beyond rape and assault situations. It enables you to hold your ground against an aggressive panhandler, obnoxious date, snooping co-worker, or inconsiderate relative; anyone, indeed, who fails to treat you with respect.

Keep in mind that boundaries vary from person to person. One woman might welcome a pat on the back from a male colleague; another might find that overly familiar. One woman might be flattered when a stranger tells her she's "lookin' good"; another might find that offensive. Therefore, it's important to know your own boundaries: what you'll tolerate and what you won't, what's appropriate for you and what isn't. Remember: unless you're aware of your own boundaries, it's difficult to respond when those boundaries are crossed.

Take the classic scenario of two teens on a date. Sometime during the evening, the boy attempts to get closer: he speaks suggestively, or his hands begin to roam. The girl is startled; she's caught off guard. She isn't immediately sure if she feels comfortable with this or not. She's never thought about her boundaries before; therefore, she says nothing. This lack of communication is a contributing factor in many date rapes.

We tend to scoff at those girls from the 1950s who insisted, "No kisses on the first date." Such pronouncements now seem as prim and dated as poodle skirts and Doris Day movies. But those girls *did* have the right idea: they had a strong sense of what their boundaries were, and they communicated them clearly.

Once you have a clear sense of your own boundaries, you're ready for the next step: protecting them with assertiveness. As any cop will tell you, burglars tend to avoid houses with alarm systems or guard dogs, favoring those that look easier to enter. It's the same for harassers or rapists. They rarely go looking for a fight; they prefer an easy score or conquest. They look for a victim likely to put up the very least resistance.

In many ways, this action is instinctive. In the wild, hungry lions will make a preemptive charge towards a herd of zebras and panic them into running. This allows them to spot those animals which lag behind, or appear old or injured. The lions then regroup and target the weakest animal.

In order to size up a potential victim, an aggressor, too, will look for signs of weakness by testing your personal boundaries. He may do so with a stare, question, comment, or joke. He may stand too close, brush against you, or put an arm around your shoulders. If you react in a startled, shocked, frightened, or complacent manner, it suggests that you may be an easy score. The same is true if you use defensive body language: avoiding eye contact, ducking your head, quickening your step, or physically retreating. An aggressor looks for the person who will fail his "test," someone who appears confused, helpless, vulnerable, intimidated, or simply passive.

At other times, an aggressor may test your boundaries in a nonaggressive manner, using a compliment or pick-up line to "reel you in." A number of years ago I received a letter from Claire, a woman whom I'd met at one of my corporate workshops. She described the following experience:

Within 24 hours of completing your workshop, I had an opportunity to test my newfound awareness. I was walking down the street when a man sitting in a parked car tried to lure me over by leaning across the passenger seat and calling out, "Do you have the time?" Without breaking stride, one quick glance in his direction told me that this wasn't someone I wanted to get within 10 feet of. I thought to myself, "Mister, you must be kidding," and I continued to ignore him. Sure enough, I could hear him shouting all kinds of obscenities as I walked away.

I was brought up in the Deep South, and for as far back as I can remember, I was taught never to be rude to anyone. Now that my safety has become my highest priority, I know I have the right to evaluate each situation and choose not to respond in accordance with outdated gender role conditioning.

In this example, Claire listened to her intuition, her inner voice. It told her that this man was someone to be avoided, that his "innocent" question was really a test of her boundaries. She responded assertively without saying a word or breaking her stride.

Remember: when an aggressor tests your boundaries, he's testing your power. Therefore, it's imperative to respond assertively the moment someone tests or violates your boundaries. Appearing strong and confident sends the message that you are in control, that you refuse to be a victim. Chances are good that your aggressor will move on to another, more accommodating victim. The last thing he wants is a struggle or a scene.

Assertiveness means expressing your feelings in a direct and honest way. And assertively protecting your boundaries does far more than defuse dangerous situations: it's a strengthening, liberating experience.

3
VERBAL EMPOWERMENT

As valuable as they are, physical techniques always involve some risk; therefore, they should be viewed as an "insurance policy" to use only in emergencies. Non-physical techniques still remain your first line of defense. In this chapter, we'll be exploring some of the ways in which words and body language can be combined to both empower and protect you.

The Art of De-Escalation

Have you ever had an encounter with someone that escalated into a yelling match? That started calmly, then turned angry, volatile, or downright ugly? Most of us have. Maybe you felt the other person wasn't listening to you, so you raised your voice to get your point across. He raised his, and before you knew it, things got out of hand. You began reacting to his anger and his emotion to the exclusion of everything else.

Anytime you react, you allow the other person to dictate the momentum and outcome of the exchange; when you act, however, it's you who takes control. And if you want to protect yourself in a volatile confrontation, taking control is a must. It's what the art of de-escalation is all about. De-escalation truly is an art form. On a daily basis, it can be used to defuse arguments and confrontations, to calm another person and "talk him down." In more threat-ening circumstances, it can prevent an actual physical assault.

In a confrontation, de-escalation helps you find that middle ground between acting too passively and too aggressively. If you act too passively, you empower your aggressor. If you act too aggressively, you may anger him and escalate the situation into violence. Men are especially guilty of the latter. Too often, their sense of macho bravado prompts them to react aggressively and escalate minor disagreements into all-out brawls.

I remember hearing from a woman just a few days after she'd attended one of my seminars. She'd been on a date and was saying good night to the man outside her door. When she didn't invite him inside, he started getting sore about it. He blocked her from entering her apartment. This angered her, and her first temptation was to raise her voice and order him to leave. But her intuition told her that this would only make things worse. She could see that he was emotional, probably because he'd had too much to drink.

So she decided to try de-escalation. She held her ground, remained calm, and quietly but firmly talked him down. Placing objectivity over pride, she stroked his ego, promising to call him the next day (yeah, right). Above all, she didn't let him see that she was intimidated. She didn't apologize, make excuses, or back away. And it worked. The man eventually ran out of steam and shuffled off.

Police officers use de-escalation all the time—and they're armed! Author George J. Thompson, Ph.D., was once a cop on the beat. In his book, *Verbal Judo,* he provides numerous examples of how he used de-escalation on the job to resolve potentially violent confrontations. In fact, he believes that the 1991 Rodney King beating could have been peacefully resolved if the officers had been better trained in de-escalation techniques.

I'll never forget watching a true-life documentary in which two officers had to intercede in a domestic dispute. The husband was waving a baseball bat and threatening to use it on his wife, on the cops, on everyone. The officers could have yelled at him to put the bat down "or else." Two against one, they might have overpowered him, or they could even have drawn their weapons.

Instead, they opted for de-escalation. Calmly yet firmly, they talked to the man: "We know you're angry but this isn't the way to handle this . . . put the bat down . . . no one's going to hurt you." And so on. Eventually, they pacified him to the point where he gave up the bat.

You don't need to be a police officer to use de-escalation. You can use it with a man or with a woman. You can use it with a stranger or with someone you know. You can use it with a spouse, co-worker, or customer. It's an excellent technique to use when the other person is emotional (angry, frustrated, out of control), or under the influence of drugs or alcohol. Keep in mind, it takes two people to have an argument. Once you refuse to participate, the other person is left with nothing to fuel his fire.

Like assertiveness, de-escalation can be used in many different situations. It works particularly well on small children, who (as any parent will tell you) often find it hard to get a grip on their emotions. I recall being at a park when two small boys got into a fistfight. Their parents quickly intervened. One father reacted emotionally, shouting at his son and grabbing his arm. By contrast, the other father remained calm. Getting down on one knee, he looked his son in the eye while disciplining him softly yet emphatically: "I know that you're upset . . . yes, I understand . . . but I will not allow this." His son eventually ran out of steam, much like that bat-wielding husband I described earlier. He regained his composure and went back to playing, the incident forgotten.

The other boy's reaction was altogether different. Though cowed by his father's outburst, he remained angry and upset. Chances were good he'd vent that anger on another child before the day was through. As you can see, one father de-escalated the situation, while the other made things worse.

De-escalation is an easy skill to learn, and the following tips will help you to develop it:

Tip #1: Don't antagonize. Don't argue, threaten, or raise your voice. Don't use obscenities or give him ultimatums. On the other hand, don't ignore him, either.

Frequently, my workshop participants will follow all these rules and *say* the right things, only to use antagonizing body language. Without realizing it, students will mirror their adversary's aggressive mannerisms by clenching their fists or taking some other antagonistic posture.

I call this "matching," and matching your aggressor's demeanor and body language will undermine any attempt at de-escalation. Although it is a totally natural response when you are threatened, it will undercut your calming words. So don't tense up; avoid clenching your fists or gritting your teeth. Don't threaten the other person physically, either by standing too close or adopting a fighting stance. And don't try to look tough and aggressive by sneering, narrowing your eyes, or jutting out your chin. Instead, keep your facial expression relaxed. Keep your hands free with your palms open towards him. In earlier times, this demonstrated that a person was unarmed; today, it's known as the universal symbol for peace.

Tip #2: Listen. Listening is a skill that can't be overestimated. When faced with someone who's emotional or out of control, listening is imperative. Try to listen—*really* listen—to what he or she is saying. Ask yourself, what does this person want from me? What's his problem? Is he simply blowing off steam, or does he want to cause me bodily harm?

Failure to listen will only antagonize the other person. Let's face it, nothing is more frustrating than talking to someone and feeling that you are not getting through. So don't raise your voice or interrupt. Don't cross your arms or look away; these only communicate one thing: I'm not listening to you! Instead, respond with phrases like, "I hear you" or "I understand"; this is known in psychology circles as "active listening." Keep your comments brief and to the point. Be firm, yet sincere, and don't patronize him.

Keep one thing in mind: active listening doesn't mean trying to see things his way. It's not about sympathizing with your aggressor, but about giving the appearance of sympathy. This will help to defuse his anger and keep the situation under your control.

Tip #3: Look for warning signs. If someone is yelling at you or shaking his fist in your face, you don't need me to tell you that he may be ready to explode. But warning signs may not always be so obvious. For example, he may be speaking calmly but his fists are clenched, or he may be silent but moving closer. Watch for these and other danger signs like sweating, rapid blinking, reddening of his face, arm waving, or looking "through" you. Listen for protracted silences, fumbling for words, or increases in the speed or volume of his voice. All can be clues that it's time to try de-escalation, or that de-escalation isn't working and you need to switch tactics.

Tip #4: Show no fear. Whatever you may be feeling inside, it's what you show on the outside that counts, so hold your ground. Don't step back or look away. Take a couple of deep breaths then speak slowly and evenly, keeping your voice calm and low. Maintain eye contact without staring.

Tip #5: Communicate clearly. Make it clear what you do or do not want: "Let go of my arm," "Step aside," and so on. You can open with empathy ("I understand that you're upset . . .") but always end with a definite statement (". . . but I want you to *leave.*").

Tip #6: Remain objective. Sometimes, remaining calm in the face of another person's anger can feel an awful lot like backing down, while matching anger with anger—giving as good as you get—can seem the stronger, more admirable response. But de-escalation is never about backing down, giving up, or surrendering control. By remaining objective, you maintain control, manipulating the situation to your advantage.

Your ego and pride are your own worst enemies in a confrontation. They get in the way of clear thinking by clouding your judgment and common sense. Ego and pride can set off a power struggle for dominance. So set them aside; try to distance yourself emotionally. Remember, de-escalation is a safety tool, no more, no less. Your aim is not to dominate the other person or win the argument, but to turn down the heat and stop verbal confrontations from boiling into physical ones. And the more skilled you are at de-escalating confrontations, the less likely you are to need your self-defense training.

Once you understand that your safety is all that really matters, you'll find it easier to remain objective.

Tip #7: Position yourself. As effective as de-escalation can be, it doesn't always work. Despite your calming words, the other person may actually get physical. To be prepared for this, your stance should be relaxed yet alert. Keep your feet shoulder-width apart to give you stability. Stay at least two arm's lengths away from your aggressor. Don't stand directly in front of him, but slightly to his left or right. This makes it harder for him to grab, shove, or strike you and provides an advantage if you choose to run or fight.

Tip #8: Remember your other options. De-escalation demands patience and perseverance; sometimes it can take time to calm a person down. But if you reach a point where you feel it isn't going to work, don't be afraid to try another approach. You'll lose none of your power in the process.

Verbal Self-Defense

There are times when taking a more forceful, direct, and aggressive approach is the best way to handle a threatening situation. That's why you need to know how to use verbal self-defense. Like de-escalation, verbal self-defense combines boundary setting, assertiveness, and body language. However, it's a less diplomatic tactic than others, with the emphasis on *you* becoming the intimidator. It's designed to put your aggressor on the defensive.

Like any other strategy, verbal self-defense should be used when your intuition tells you it's called for. It's most effective when you sense that an aggressor will be surprised by your actions. Here's a good example of it in practice:

> *A woman is followed by a stranger as she walks towards her car. As he gets closer, she turns and faces him with her shoulders squared and her legs apart. She looks him in the eye, takes a step forward, and orders him, "Back off! Now!"*

This woman is guided by her intuition. She feels that by appearing strong and confident, and seizing the initiative, she's more likely to attract public attention and put *him* on the defensive. That's what verbal self-defense is all about. Don't shy away from using powerful commands to get your message across. "No," "Back off," "Get lost," and "Don't even think about it," are all examples of powerful and direct commands.

Here are the rules of Verbal Self-Defense:

1. Take a step *forward*.
2. Use short, to-the-point commands. These can include profanity, but your commands can be just as forceful without it.
3. Leave no room for discussion. Don't answer his questions or try to justify yourself.
4. Back up your message with appropriate body language.
5. Be ready for his next move.
6. SHOW NO FEAR.

There's always the possibility that your aggressor may ignore your command to "Back off!" He may step closer or continue talking to you. If this happens, take another step forward and repeat your command louder and stronger: "I told you to back off!" Extend your arms towards him at eye level, as if to say, "Stop right there!"

Don't step back, look away, or turn your back on him to leave. Don't get drawn into a dialogue. Keep your commands short and to the point, and continue to repeat them until he does what you want him to do.

And keep in mind that you do have other options. You can hail a cab, duck into a crowd of people, or walk up to other people and tell them what's happening. (They don't have to get involved; just the appearance of aligning yourself with others can discourage an aggressor.) If he keeps following you, you can get to a phone and call the police. If he blocks you from leaving or lays a hand on you, you can fight.

Aleisha, a young woman living in San Francisco, had an experience that perfectly illustrates the importance and effectiveness of verbal self-defense.

Leaving her office after work, just months after taking an assertiveness training course, Aleisha was in a crowded elevator when she felt a hand brush against her thigh. She immediately turned towards the man who touched her and told him loudly and forcefully to keep his "goddamn hands" to himself. Everyone in the elevator was taken aback, including the harasser. Hotly denying Aleisha's accusation, he tried to put her on the defensive: "What's your problem, lady?" But Aleisha held her ground and came back again with "Keep your hands off me!" When the elevator reached the lobby, the man dashed out of the building.

A few weeks later, another woman was also targeted in downtown San Francisco by a man who repeatedly touched and rubbed against her in an office elevator. When she didn't rebuff those violations, he followed her out of the building and raped her. Arrested soon afterward, this rapist turned out to be—you guessed it—the same man who had fondled Aleisha.

As I've said before, an attacker looks for people who appear unsure of themselves, oblivious to their surroundings, anxious, frightened, and powerless. He makes the well-founded assumption that an individual who fails to fight back verbally is less likely to fight back physically. That's why verbal self-defense must be understood and mastered *prior* to learning physical self-defense. The verbal always supports the physical.

Like any other technique, verbal self-defense has its limitations. Let's say, for example, that an aggressor has confronted you in a seemingly isolated location, with no one else within earshot. In this situation, your command to "Back off!" may fall on deaf ears. But while he may not be deterred by it, *you still lose nothing by trying verbal self-defense*. It may work. And because it replaces reaction with action, it will energize and empower you if you do make the choice to fight.

Verbal self-defense is most effective when other people are around or may be close by. It draws attention to an aggressor or harasser, and attention is the very last thing he wants. It also sends the message that you will not be complacent: when you're verbally assertive, it suggests that you're prepared to protect yourself physically if you need to.

In my experience, people are often reluctant to use verbal self-defense because they fear it will anger an aggressor and therefore put them in greater danger. However, appearing weak or passive rarely discourages an attack, while verbal self-defense can and often does. And while it obviously helps if you have the fighting skills to back up your words, don't let the fact that you're elderly, frail, or otherwise physically handicapped stop you from employing verbal self-defense. Depending on the situation, it may be your very best option. I was reminded of this one day as I rode in an elevator with two very elderly women. It occurred to me that if I'd been an attacker, I would have had them trapped. And I couldn't help but think, "These women are so frail . . . how could they physically defend themselves? They have trouble just *walking* on their own!" It struck me then that verbal self-defense would be their best means of protection against an attacker. At the very least, it might buy them some time, catch an attacker off guard, and attract the attention of others.

As with any self-defense technique, there are no hard and fast rules about when and where to use verbal self-defense. No two situations are alike, so let your intuition guide you. Even in a situation where you have made the choice to fight, for example, your intuition might be telling you to forget the assertive approach and feign helplessness instead; this can lure your aggressor into a false sense of security and give you the advantage of surprise.

Note: One mistake that many people make when employing verbal resistance is coupling their command with a warning. They say, "Back off or I'll hurt you," or "Get out of my way or I'll fight." Don't do this! Warnings have no, repeat *no* place in the self-defense equation. You want surprise to be on your side anytime you choose to fight. Also, warnings can antagonize an aggressor; telling someone, "Back off or I'll hurt you" sounds like a challenge and is more likely to provoke an attack than deter one. You have the right to take action if someone blocks you, corners you, or lays a hand on you, and you have no reason—or obligation—to warn him first.

Meanwhile, don't underestimate the power of verbal self-defense. It can and does work in many situations. Once you refuse to be a victim of anyone's harassment or threats, you're halfway home.

Moving in the Right Direction: The Power of Stepping Forward

Most of us are accustomed to stepping back when someone enters our personal space. Sometimes this is just good manners, as when we make room for others in a crowded elevator. More often, it's an instinctive response when our physical boundaries are violated. Yet this same response will undermine any verbal resistance strategy. It signals fear and weakness to an aggressor, something you never want to do.

Step forward and you retain your power. Step backward or step aside and you give your power away. It's that simple. It's no use ordering an aggressor to "Back off!" if you're backing away as you say it. You're sending a mixed message: the words are there, but the body language implies a lack of conviction. As I stated earlier, body language is more powerful than the spoken word. It's crucial that you hold your ground and deliver your message with power and confidence. Stepping forward makes this possible.

Keep one thing in mind: don't step forward with just one foot, leaving your other foot behind. Always stand squarely on both feet when facing an aggressor.

I recall the account of one of my Boston students who, after exiting a subway, was approached by an unsavory character with a bad attitude. Recalling her training, she turned towards him, took that all-important step forward, and delivered some choice words not fit to print! It worked like a charm. Put it all together. Step forward and assertively deliver your message. That's how you retain your power.

The best way to master this strategy is to incorporate it into your daily life. The next time you find yourself in a friendly dialogue, take a step forward and see what happens. Chances are, your listener will register mild surprise, but he'll pay more attention to what you have to say. But if you're locked in a confrontation, stepping forward can shift the balance of power in your favor. Your listener may even take a step back. You'll find yourself feeling more confident and empowered. And with time, you'll begin stepping forward naturally and instinctively whenever the situation calls for it.

* * *

Never underestimate the effectiveness of verbal techniques like de-escalation and verbal self-defense. I have yet to meet the woman who didn't feel more confident and empowered after learning these essential skills. And now that you have learned them, you too can enjoy the sense of greater freedom and control over your life that these tools most assuredly offer.

4

THE PSYCHOLOGY OF EMPOWERMENT

The Power Within: Creating Your Own Reality

"Power tools" like assertiveness and intuition will empower you, and so will techniques like verbal self-defense. And yet there is nothing quite so strong as the empowerment that comes from within. "What's the key to self-empowerment?" is a question I'm asked all the time by workshop participants looking for an edge. And my answer is simple: self-empowerment is a creation of your own reality.

When I began studying the martial arts in 1986, I never thought for a minute that I'd achieve black belt ranking. It was so far from my reality that I didn't even consider it a possibility. I would watch the black belts train, but always with the conviction that they were in a class by themselves, a class that Al Marrewa could never be a part of.

I set a limited reality for myself in other aspects of my life as well. If some goals were attainable, some never would be. I placed a wall, a dividing line, around my expectations and dreams. Worse yet, I rationalized that my attitude was practical and realistic. In fact, I was selling myself short.

That way of thinking had become my standard operating procedure. I'd created a reality where achievement in any arena—martial arts or otherwise—was going to be virtually impossible. Needless to say, my martial arts training suffered because of the "reality" in which I lived. And so did my work, and my relationships. It wasn't until I experienced a personal disaster in 1989—a brief marriage that ended in divorce—that I decided to take control of my life once and for all. With the help of a professional counselor, I gained new insight into the attitudes, behaviors, and personal choices that had shaped my life up to that point. I learned that I was in no small measure responsible for the direction my life had taken, and that I alone had the power to change that direction. Over time, I began to find more success in my work, and I developed more healthy personal relationships. Creating a new reality for myself, a reality filled with opportunity and higher goals, was an important part of that process.

Talking to my students, I've heard them describe their own walls, those boundaries they've erected around their dreams and expectations. One woman aspired to get her supervisor's job, but felt that her aspiration was just plain unrealistic. Another thought it foolhardy to think that she could ever double or triple her current salary. Their stories are typical. It's easy for all of us to create a reality that shortchanges our very future.

All too often we let other people determine our own reality. We wait for *them* to tell us that we can reach our goals; we wait for their encouragement. Unfortunately, that encouragement doesn't always materialize. Empowerment from without—from the praise, approval, and sanction of other people—is often long in coming, if it comes at all. Self-empowerment, on the other hand, is always within your reach. You have the ability to create your own reality, a reality in which this personal strength becomes not just a possibility, but a probability.

Creating your own reality means different things to different people. For some women who enroll in my program, it means empowering themselves physically; for others, it means becoming more assertive. Some students want to stop being afraid of living alone, while others want to establish healthy personal relationships where dignity and mutual respect are not the exception but the rule.

As students enter my program for the first time, I urge them to examine their current reality or world. Does that reality include the idea of full personal empowerment? If it doesn't, their very first task is to create a new reality for themselves.

This same mind-set is for you and you alone to create. Even if you can't change the whole world, the power to change *your* world is always within your grasp.

Victimhood versus Personhood: The Choice Is Yours

At the risk of angering many people, I believe that the concept of "victimhood" is one of the greatest societal ills of today. Simply stated, seeing yourself as a victim only ensures that you will remain one.

From the beginning of time, men have treated women as property, as an owned and coveted commodity. A complete reversal in this way of thinking has been slow in coming. The progress that American women have achieved in the last century has been impressive, yet total balance between the sexes has yet to be achieved, and may never be realized in our lifetimes. Even today, violence against women is all too common. So is discrimination. Logically speaking, women should never be described as a "minority" since they make up over half the population. Like racial minorities, however, they've encountered a disproportionate share of discrimination. But if the world never balances out, you as an individual can still bring balance to *your* world. This is done by choosing personhood over victimhood.

It's all too easy for us to blame others for our own misfortunes, failures, and unfulfilled dreams. Playing the victim can even be rewarding in the short term, bringing you sympathy and attention from others. Yet victimhood is the proverbial dead-end street. As long as you see yourself as a victim, you will lack the power to accomplish the goals you wish to achieve.

Over the years, I've met many women who were targets of violent crime. They could easily (and understandably) see themselves as victims. Instead, they choose to see themselves as survivors. These women remain a constant inspiration to me. Violence has touched their lives and forever changed them, yet they have opted for personhood over victimhood.

Victimhood is the antithesis of personal empowerment. In the excellent *What You Feel, You Can Heal* by John Gray, Ph.D., he describes a Victim as someone who usually feels powerless. He goes on to say that the Victim refuses to take responsibility for her life and sucks others into trying to please her and make her happy.

Deep-seated, repressed anger is another element of victimhood: anger about failure, about disappointment, about "fate" that manifests itself in resentment and envy of others. An angry person is, at the core, angry at herself. By contrast, the empowered person loves herself and is able to approach others in an equally positive way.

There will always be men who place women in the role of victims whenever they can. Part of this has to do with the discomfort they feel around powerful, self-assured women. Competent, capable, empowered women threaten their masculine identity. Take note: this is their problem, not yours. No one's opinion should determine your reality. Exercise your power by playing your game, not theirs. This applies to survival on the street, at the office, at home, and anywhere else that falls under the umbrella of "your world."

Self-Esteem in the Empowerment Equation

In the late 1980s, many educators broke away from traditional thinking and began to focus on the psychological needs of school-age children. Their research demonstrated a direct link between low self-esteem and such psychological and emotional problems as substance abuse, eating disorders, and violence in the classroom. In some schools, this led to the introduction of separate self-esteem curricula.

As any psychologist will tell you, your level of self-esteem is part and parcel of who you are. It has a direct impact on how you function on a daily basis: how you make decisions, relate to others, and deal with conflict.

High self-esteem is the thread that holds together all of my concepts and ideas on personal empowerment. It's that important. Furthermore, it's an essential component of assault prevention:

the woman who refuses to see herself as a potential victim is far less likely to become one.

There's also a marvelous link between self-esteem and physical self-defense. High self-esteem will enhance your ability to defend yourself and learning self-defense will bolster your self-esteem. Each feeds the other, and neither works in isolation. By way of illustration, let's use the analogy of two boxers before a championship fight. Boxer A is favored to win: he's an experienced fighter with many victories to his credit, and he has incredible talent and skill. But while Boxer A has worked his way up the ranks, defeating boxers with less skill and ability, he doesn't believe in himself. He's plagued by self-doubt. His self-esteem is low.

By contrast, Boxer B *does* believe in himself. Though less talented than his opponent, Boxer B's confidence and winning attitude have convinced him that he will emerge triumphant. And if I was putting money on their fight, I'd bet the farm on Boxer B! I'd take self-confidence, self-respect, and a positive attitude over talent, ability, and low self-esteem any time.

Time and time again, I've seen women with high self-esteem become skilled at self-defense with very little training. How can this be? Because technique and ability are secondary. It's more important that you love, respect, and believe in yourself. Only then will you be ready to do what it takes to protect yourself.

No amount of physical training will empower you if you see yourself as a victim. That's true whether you're a man or a woman, and whether you're five-foot-two or six-foot-three. You may be a "Mack truck" but you can't go anywhere without an engine, and high self-esteem is that engine. Without it, you'll never get out of first gear. High self-esteem makes you believe, "I am worth fighting for, and I *will* succeed." In an assault situation, it will enable you to fight with determination, focus, and 100 percent commitment. In your daily life, it will drive you towards any goal you wish to achieve.

Levels of self-esteem vary from person to person. However, it doesn't matter where you start, what matters is where you're headed. You're in the driver's seat. You might need a backseat driver or two—a teacher, counselor, or therapist—but the power is in your hands. If life's true meaning is found not in the destination but in the journey, your journey can start now, and you have an entire lifetime to reach your goal.

Personal empowerment means so much more than knowing self-defense. The vast majority of my students have never found themselves in an assault situation, but none of them feel that their empowerment training was a waste of time. Why? Because it's given them a strength, confidence, and self-respect that has affected every area of their lives.

Looking Within: The Value of Self-Assessment

When I first began teaching personal empowerment, I focused primarily on the techniques of self-defense. Over time, however, I began to notice that while certain women were able to apply the most elaborate techniques with ease, others struggled with even the most basic concepts. It made no difference if they were young or old, tall or petite, fit or out of shape. Clearly, some other factor was at work.

I realized that my approach was missing a vital component, a component that could either make or break an otherwise sound empowerment program. It became clear to me that our response to confrontation, as well as our very attitudes towards verbal and physical self-defense, are largely determined by our previous life experiences.

I began to ask students to look back on their lives and identify experiences that might have had a particular impact on their self-image. Some of them found this easy. One woman remembered a gym teacher telling her she was "uncoordinated"; she spent the rest of her life assuming this was true. Another recalled her mother's admonishment that "Nice girls do not fight." Yet another remembered the humiliation of scuffling with a boy her age and being easily overpowered. On the positive side, some women attributed the confidence they had in their physical abilities to the fact that they'd been tomboys growing up, or were "always good at sports."

Still other women confessed to seeing themselves as timid, weak, or incompetent, but couldn't understand the reasons why. They had to dig deeper to identify the life experiences which had contributed to that self-image.

Although adult experiences *do* contribute to one's psychological and emotional makeup, I've found that those from childhood and adolescence have a far more lasting impact. As children, we're particularly influenced by parents, siblings, and role models such as teachers; as teenagers, we're more influenced by our peers. Furthermore, our self-image is affected by how we see girls and women—and boys and men—portrayed on television and in the movies. Even in today's supposedly more liberated times, women on film are routinely portrayed as victims: as passive, helpless, or overly emotional. Men take action, women wait on the sidelines; it's an all too familiar scenario. Finally, our self-image is affected by our personal traumas and successes.

All of these influences and experiences affect your ability to take action when faced with a confrontation, life-threatening or otherwise. To paraphrase one of my instructors, "You bring all your baggage to a fight."

Do you find it hard to stand up for yourself, either verbally or physically? If so, ask yourself why. Identify any particular fears, insecurities, inhibitions, or anything else that might be holding you back from achieving true empowerment.

For some people, this self-assessment may be a fairly easy process. It may be as simple as telling oneself, "I'm not the child I was; I'm an adult now and I have the power to change my self-image." For others, professional therapy may be needed to help them understand the deeper issues that act as roadblocks. Remember, those who bring too much "baggage" to a fight stand a good chance of losing, so try to travel light!

Power comes in many forms: mental, emotional and physical, just to name a few. When I ask men to assess what makes them "powerful," most include their physicality. For most women, however, physicality hasn't traditionally been a part of their sense of personal power. Yet I believe that knowing how to physically defend yourself is an essential component of inner strength. It's a liberating form of empowerment that will have an impact on many other areas of your life. It *does* require a commitment that, quite frankly, most people are not willing to make. But if you do make that commitment, you'll learn much more than how to protect yourself: you'll tap into your true potential as a human being. Through my training, I've seen women acquire compassion, perspective, objectivity, balance, discipline, and confidence. As a testament to the emotional and spiritual benefits that this kind of training has to offer, here are some excerpts from letters I've received over the years:

"It's given me a sense of power and self-esteem that is overwhelming. I love feeling in control."

"I no longer see myself as a five-foot-three, 105-pound weakling: I am a small fury."

"I now realize that I can be assertive without it meaning that I'm a cold-hearted 'bitch.'"

"I can now be polite and assertive at the same time. I even won an argument at work."

"I was left with such a strong feeling of myself."

"I feel so much more comfortable living my life."

"I've learned new ways to make decisions."

"I feel like a completely new person."

"The strength I've acquired has enabled me to be more compassionate towards everyone in my life."

Say It, Hear It, Believe It: The Power of Positive "Self-Talk"

Negative talk is something that we're all too familiar with. We've all been criticized, sometimes harshly. Since childhood, even well-meaning parents, relatives, teachers, and friends have reminded us of our limitations. Sometimes we believe these negative messages to such an extent that they harm our self-image. And a negative self-image not only stops you from learning, growing, and achieving your full potential as a human being: it makes you a less-than-formidable foe to an abuser, harasser, or attacker.

So how do you break away from low self-concept and destructive self-criticism? One answer is **positive self-talk.** Through positive self-talk, you reinforce positive messages about who you are and what you're capable of accomplishing. Depending on others for these positive messages isn't enough; indeed, they may never come. When positive messages come from within, however, you control the reshaping of your own self-image. Even if you feel your self-image is pretty healthy to begin with, positive self-talk will only enhance it.

Positive self-talk is a way of talking to yourself. You silently repeat simple yet powerful affirmations of who you are as a human being and what you will accomplish. For example, "I deserve to be loved," is an affirmation, while positive self-talk is the vehicle by which that affirmation is reinforced, again and again, until it becomes a part of your self-image. You may affirm your value as a person ("I am a strong and capable woman"), your capabilities ("I have the power to reach my goals"), or what you are entitled to ("I deserve to be happy").

One simple yet effective idea is to write down selected affirmations on index cards (one per card), then post them around your home. Your affirmations can be general, or specific ("This week, I will be more assertive"). Each time you come across a card, read what it says, then silently repeat it once or twice. Better yet, repeat it aloud; this will only give it more impact.

Dan Millman, former world champion gymnast and author of *The Warrior Athlete,* writes of low self-concept and destructive self-criticism as two key contributors to failure on and off the playing field. Quite frankly, you can have all the talent and skill in the world, yet never achieve success if you don't say it, hear it, and believe it.

Next time you watch a boxing match on television, listen to the trainer coaching his fighter between rounds. Sometimes he offers fighting tips; just as often, he focuses on the boxer's morale. He gives encouragement. He knows his boxer will not win the match unless he believes in himself and his abilities.

With positive self-talk, you become your own coach. In the end, the encouragement and affirmations you need to triumph over any obstacle must come from within. And that's true no matter who you are. As knowledgeable as many martial artists are about self-defense, for example, many would actually be in big trouble if attacked. Self-doubt, low self-esteem, and destructive self-criticism would inhibit their ability to fight as surely as any physical handicap. I would have more confidence in the abilities of a person who'd learned just *one* fighting technique and had a positive self-image than I would in a black belt who was plagued with self-doubt.

The use of positive self-talk is directly related to the concept of creating your own reality, described earlier. Creating your own reality begins with how you see yourself. With a healthy self-image reinforced by positive affirmations, *you* become the "energy source" that will drive you towards a more fulfilling and meaningful life.

At the same time, try to surround yourself with people who maintain a positive outlook on life. People who are negative—especially those who tend to criticize and judge you—will do nothing but harm to your self-image. In my opinion, they should be given permanent exit passes out of your life! Of course, you may not be able to eliminate every negative person from your life. Some family ties, for example, are better left unbroken. But whenever possible, examine your relationships, long-standing or otherwise. Ask yourself, "Does this person make me feel like a special human being? Does he or she have a positive influence on my life?" If the answer is no, take steps to either change or end that relationship. All too often, fear of change or simple force of habit keeps us in relationships that are no longer healthy or beneficial.

I can give one example of this from my own life. Bob was a fraternity brother and close friend of mine from college. But if people change—sometimes for the better, sometimes for the worse—so do friendships. As the years went by, I saw Bob acquire a deeply negative outlook on people, the world, on life itself. It took me a while to realize that his negativity was threatening my own positive outlook. Friendships should give us support, encouragement, and strength, helping us to be better human beings. At some point, my friendship with Bob stopped giving me any of these things; in fact, it made me feel more cynical and pessimistic. It had lasted for years, but was now doing me far more harm than good. So, on my initiative, we eventually parted company. Life is challenging enough without the burden of others' negativity. Relationships with people who are positive about life and positive about you will only strengthen your own self-image.

The idea behind positive self-talk is that if you say it and hear it, you will eventually believe it. Once you start telling yourself, "Personal empowerment *is* within my grasp," you're on the road to making it a reality.

You may be skeptical that positive self-talk can really be so powerful, or is really that important. You might be thinking that practical techniques like de-escalation or self-defense are all that truly matter. Yet techniques alone will never be enough: while they will give you more confidence in your ability to protect yourself, true confidence really must come from within. Towards the end of their training, I ask students, "Do you believe that you'll respond assertively if you're threatened, harassed, or physically assaulted? Will you be able to respond with 100 percent commitment?" If they answer "I hope so," or "I'd like to think so," their training isn't completed.

With repeated positive self-talk, your self-image will vastly improve. You're more likely to find success: not only in an assault situation, but in all other areas of your life. Never forget that you alone have the power to change anything!

Maintaining Your Perspective: The Importance of Objectivity

As I define it, objectivity is the ability to see people, situations, and experiences for what they really are. It means distancing yourself from emotions that tend to cloud your judgment.

By the time you finish reading this book, you will have learned many different strategies. These strategies will help you handle everything from minor confrontations to violent assault, and each and every one of them depends on objectivity. Objectivity allows you to assess situations and respond appropriately; in an assault situation, it's as much a fighting technique as an elbow in the ribs or a slap to the testicles. And just as importantly, learning to remain objective will help you in your daily life.

Emotions are the greatest obstacle to objectivity, especially the emotions of anger and fear. Stepping back from these emotions allows you to see people and situations with greater clarity. Is this always possible? Is complete objectivity a realistic goal? Of course not, unless you're Mr. Spock! We're human beings, not robots; we can't remain rational and unemotional in every situation, confrontational or otherwise. But simply aiming for objectivity will bring you many unexpected benefits.

Let me offer you one example of this. While standing in a line at the DMV, I noticed that the man ahead of me was angry and impatient. As he reached the head of the line, he exploded at the woman behind the counter. He was loud and threatening, his language abusive. All heads turned in his direction; a showdown seemed inevitable.

Then the unexpected happened. The DMV clerk appeared to mentally "step back" from the confrontation, as if reasoning, "This man's not really angry at me. He's angry at something else, and I'm going to try to find out what that is." In other words, she remained objective. She was only human and it couldn't have been easy for her to endure such verbal abuse. But she managed to overlook his insults and listen to his complaint. In the end, she came up with a solution acceptable to both parties. The situation didn't get out of control. She "kept the customer happy" because she was able to judge his complaint not on its delivery, but on its merits.

I used to look at people and make quick, conclusive judgments. I didn't view people objectively, but through a cloud of personal biases, prejudices, and attitudes. What's more, I wasn't even aware that I was doing this. When I brought this mind-set to the martial arts studio, I learned that my lack of objectivity put me at greater risk on the street. Let's say, for example, that you are confronted by an armed robber in an underground garage. Lacking objectivity, your reaction may be determined by pure emotion: fear (you panic and freeze), outrage (you refuse his demands for money), or anger (you try to fight him off). As a result, you may be shot and even killed. Objectivity might have prevented this. It would have helped you to think more clearly and weigh your options and choices.

Even in situations where you choose to fight back, you must assess your opponent and the situation objectively. Emotion will inhibit you from doing either. Muhammad Ali knew this, and used it in the ring. Time and again, he'd provoke his opponent with verbal taunts, insulting body language, you name it. He *wanted* his opponent to get angry, knowing that emotion would impair his opponent's ability to fight.

I can still remember when it hit me why remaining objective makes so much sense. I was at the martial arts studio, changing after an exhausting workout, when I spotted a book in my instructor's open locker. It was entitled *You Are Not the Target*. The implications of this title were a revelation: I realized that most confrontations have absolutely nothing to do with me as a person.

One day, while waiting for a friend outside his apartment, I double-parked and kept the engine running. I didn't notice when a truck drove up behind me and tried unsuccessfully to maneuver around my car. Suddenly the truck driver was pounding on my window, yelling expletives not fit to print. For one brief moment, I was tempted to bolt from my car and give it right back to him. Fortunately, my objectivity prevailed. I realized he wasn't angry at me, he just wanted me to move my car. He probably had a tight schedule to keep and I was making him late. So I moved my car and he drove on—end of story. Just because he reacted inappropriately was no reason for me to do the same.

If I'd let my emotions tell me what to do, I would have become embroiled in an argument with that driver. And by escalating the situation, I would have done more than wasted my time and energy: I might have placed myself at risk. In this day and age, it's not uncommon for drivers to carry a loaded weapon in their cars. In many situations, therefore, objectivity can quite literally save your life.

People often take out their own anger, frustration, or unhappiness on an innocent party. Think about it: have you ever lashed out at someone who just happened to be there? I know I have. More than once, I've directed my anger towards someone who had absolutely nothing to do with the source of my anger. Psychologists call this "displacement"; you may know it as "kicking the cat" because you've had a bad day.

When confronted by a person who's angry or out of control,

remember that you are not the target. Even if you said or did something that triggered his anger, that anger is *his* problem. So don't take it personally! Step back from your emotions, and you'll find it much easier to handle stressful confrontations.

Objectivity will also allow you to assess situations for what they really are. Sharon was only 18 years old when she started work as a legal secretary. Within a few months, she became the target of unwelcome sexual advances from a lawyer in her office. From both an ethical and legal standpoint, this man's behavior was clearly out of line; just as clearly, Sharon had every right to take action, either by confronting him directly, reporting him to management, or both. Unfortunately, Sharon was unable to think objectively because her emotions got in the way. The harassment made her feel so embarrassed, nervous, and confused, she began to dread going to work and eventually quit her job.

Twenty years later, Sharon is able to look back and see her ordeal for what it really was: a textbook example of sexual harassment in which she was the innocent party. She can be more objective about her experience because she is viewing it from an entirely different *perspective:* that of a now mature and sophisticated woman. In many ways, her story illustrates why perspective goes hand in hand with objectivity.

Perspective also plays a role in learning physical self-defense. My particular fighting style, Kung Fu San Soo, is a Chinese fighting system that is thousands of years old. It was created when five Chinese families combined their respective expertise in military fighting. One family contributed all types of kicks and punches, while others contributed throws, leverages, takedowns, and so on. While each family's techniques were effective on their own, pooling them created a fighting art greater than the sum of its parts.

When I teach San Soo, my students learn much more than its various techniques. They learn to approach and execute those techniques from different positions and perspectives: from the front and rear of their opponent, the left and right, from standing, seated, and ground-level positions. I want them to see every available opportunity.

If you can't see opportunities, you can't take advantage of them. I saw this principle in practice with one of my San Soo students.

Sandra was a 35-year-old financial analyst, and one of the first things I noticed about her was how bright she was. She responded best to detailed explanations of each concept and technique. This made perfect sense because she had an analytical mind. She was probably drawn to her field because that's how her mind worked best. Her kind of work requires what I call "linear thinking," and most accountants, bankers, lawyers, and technical professionals use linear thinking in their work and personal lives.

Sandra was a very good fighter. She moved well and could execute a number of techniques with incredible precision. However, San Soo requires more than mere analysis of its concepts and techniques. It requires creativity, openness and "feel." Sandra's linear mind-set made it difficult for her to master techniques based on intuition and feel. As I got to know her, I learned that Sandra also lived in a way that discouraged experimentation and creativity. It was important for her to feel in control.

Don't get me wrong: there's nothing wrong with control, but when you try to control *everything,* experimentation and creativity tend to go out the window. Linear thinkers have difficulty becoming great San Soo fighters unless they can open themselves up to new and unfamiliar perspectives. Remember: balance is the key, not only to self-defense, but to life. As someone who was once a linear thinker, I learned this lesson the hard way.

For years, I was very much like Sandra. I analyzed and tried to control my world. I had tunnel vision, and brought this rigid way of thinking to the martial arts studio. I tried to analyze and control my workout at every turn, yet I foundered when it came to instinct, intuition, and creativity. I found it hard to be flexible, preferring instead to repeat familiar patterns and habits. Because I was left-handed, for example, I favored my left with every punch or kick. I also approached my opponent from the left and attacked just one side of his body. Fortunately, my instructor was smart enough to see this, and for an entire month forced me to approach my opponent not from the left but from the right. The first time I tried it, it felt awkward and unfamiliar. With time and practice, however, I gradually mastered this approach and learned to "see" my opponent from more than one perspective. As a result, I became a more flexible and well-rounded fighter.

Parents who want to "baby-proof" their homes are often advised to get down on their hands and knees and go from room to room. Why? Because adopting the perspective of a small child will help them spot dangers they might otherwise miss. To see anything objectively, you should always try to approach it from different points of view. I was home watching television one night, for example, when I decided to pick up my chair, turn it around, and move it to a completely different part of the room. Then I sat down and looked around. The effect was dramatic. By viewing the room from an entirely new and unfamiliar perspective, I noticed things about it I had never noticed before. More importantly, this simple exercise served as a metaphor: I began to see the value of breaking out of old habits and approaching *life* from more than one perspective. I invite you to do the same: as you encounter new people, events, and situations, try to see them from different points of view. Experiment with different attitudes, beliefs, and behaviors. It won't always be easy, and it won't always feel comfortable, but sometimes you have to break out of your comfort zone to see "the big picture."

* * *

As I emphasized to you at the beginning of this chapter, personal power must ultimately come from within. And regardless of your previous life experiences, you *do* have the power to choose the direction of your life from this day forward. In the next chapter, we'll begin to explore some of the ways in which your personal power may be challenged by others. As we do so, I urge you to reject the "victim" mentality and believe in the strength you possess as a woman, and as a human being.

5

HARASSMENT: LIFE IN THE MODERN WORLD

Sexual Harassment

In 1991, the allegations by Professor Anita Hill against Supreme Court nominee Clarence Thomas captured the attention of an entire nation and put sexual harassment in the spotlight. Yet sexual harassment existed long before 1991, and it continues to be a reality of modern life that cannot be denied. Speaking for myself, I have met hundreds of women who have experienced it on the job.

Under the umbrella of "workplace harassment," there are two types of sexual harassment: quid pro quo and hostile work environment. The law provides protection from both, but makes a definite distinction between the two.

Loosely translated, quid pro quo means "one thing in return for another." This type of harassment occurs when a person in a position of power or authority demands sexual favors in exchange for an employee's job security, a promotion, or a pay increase. A hostile work environment, on the other hand, applies to any unwanted or offensive overtures, references, language, jokes, touching, or displays of photographs directed at one employee by another, regardless of either worker's position in the company. (The laws of varying states define hostile work environment as that which would offend "a reasonable woman" or "a reasonable person.")

Therefore, if your boss or employer demands sexual favors from you in return for a promotion, that's quid pro quo harassment. If a colleague hangs up a *Playboy* centerfold in plain view of your desk, that's a hostile work environment.

Many corporations have drawn up policies aimed at preventing sexual harassment in the workplace, not only to protect their workers, but also their shareholders: a sexual harassment suit can damage both a company's image and its fiscal bottom line. Comprehensive sexual harassment policies have been long overdue and they're appropriate to a setting where a woman can lose a promotion, raise, or job if she rejects a sexual advance, or has to endure a hostile workplace environment. Taken too far, however, these protective policies can reinforce a dangerous notion, the notion that women cannot take care of themselves.

In Victorian days, women were encouraged to see men as their protectors. By now suggesting that women need a bureaucracy to protect them, we risk taking one bad crutch and replacing it with another. Instead of encouraging women to communicate clearly and assertively in their personal interactions, these policies can infantilize women and encourage an over-dependence upon others. One case in point: the elaborate guidelines that some colleges have drawn up to "regulate" student dating. These dating policies attempt to codify everything from "unwelcome advances" to the meaning of "consent." Though obviously well-intentioned, I believe these kinds of guidelines do far more harm than good. They perpetuate the long-standing myth that women need special protection, that compared to men, they're less capable of communicating what they do or don't want. And by setting a one-size-fits-all definition of acceptable behavior, they don't allow for the fact that "acceptable" means different things to different people. What one woman finds flattering, another might find offensive. What one calls romantic interest, another might call harassment.

Policies and laws do have their value in certain situations, but you don't always need them to protect you. You're capable of handling many situations on your own, and I urge you to use that capability whenever and wherever you can.

I recall running into Elaine, a friend of mine who works at a health club. With some pride, Elaine said that she had just filed a sexual harassment complaint against a co-worker who had been making innuendos about her body and appearance. Elaine found them deeply offensive and wasted no time in complaining to her employer.

When I asked what *she* had said to her harasser, Elaine seemed surprised by the question. She hadn't said anything to him, and didn't intend to ("Why should I?" she asked). This was a confident young woman who was otherwise assertive in her daily life. Yet her first reaction was to have someone else take care of the problem. By doing so, she probably reinforced her harasser's opinion that women are inherently helpless, and made him feel more powerful. After all, it took the whole system, the whole bureaucracy, to put him in his place!

If Elaine had confronted that man directly, there's a good chance she might have put a stop to his innuendos right then and there. It's possible her co-worker had no idea he was making her so uncomfortable or was saying anything inappropriate; he might have apologized profusely if she'd made it clear his comments were not appreciated. And, by handling the situation herself, Elaine would have been exercising her power. Later, if the harassment continued, she still could have appealed to a higher authority.

In my experience, most inappropriate behavior can be halted immediately with a direct, assertive response. If someone's behavior offends you, confront that person yourself and there's a good chance you will stop the harassment in its tracks. And the sooner you address it, the better: the longer you wait, the more likely you are to *need* assistance from others later on. Just as importantly, trying to resolve situations yourself fosters a self-reliant attitude, and self-reliance is what personal empowerment is all about.

At the same time, try to keep things in perspective. Beware of the tendency to slap a "harassment" label on every little instance of rude, thoughtless, or adolescent behavior. Choose your battles and save your time and energy for real violations of your boundaries. If someone's behavior bothers you, try to ask yourself, "Is this behavior truly offensive to me, or is it merely irritating? Is it really worthy of my attention, or better left alone? Do I really need the assistance of others to put a stop to it, or can I handle it on my own?" Remain objective and make these decisions for yourself.

Street Harassment

If you've never been harassed while out in public, you're in the lucky minority. For most women, it's become part of modern life. While millions of women go their whole lives without ever encountering rape or assault, I have yet to meet one who hasn't endured street harassment in some form or another.

A street harasser may be an obnoxious drunk or "street crazy." He may be a panhandler who follows you down the street, or one of a gang of catcalling construction workers. He may be a stranger who makes little "kissy" sounds, or mutters some sexual remark. Or he may be someone who persists in talking to you when you just want to be left alone.

When I bring up street harassment to an audience, the room practically explodes. It touches an emotional chord; everyone has a story to tell. Clearly, street harassment is one of the most irritating things women have to deal with in public. Even in its most innocent forms—that panhandler outside the supermarket, let's say—it's the rare woman (or man) who doesn't find it stressful to some degree. I know I do. We all find it frustrating because we feel so powerless to stop it.

What transforms street harassment from being merely irritating to deeply unsettling is its underlying potential for violence. And it's true: when you're dealing with strangers on the street, you can't take anything for granted. Any situation can turn ugly. But while you should exercise caution with street harassers, you don't have to live in fear of them. You can still exercise your power.

Panhandlers

When I talk about panhandlers as a form of street harassment, I'm not referring to the genuinely needy person who quietly and politely asks you for change. I'm talking about the guy who's made panhandling his line of work and uses intimidation to get your money. The former asks for charity; the latter employs a form of extortion. If you refuse his request, he may turn insulting, obscene, or even threatening. He may step too close, brush against you, or grab your arm. He may block your way or stop you from entering your car. He may follow you down the street.

"How should I deal with aggressive panhandlers?" is a question I'm asked all the time. And my advice is, "Give them what they want." That's usually what I do. The way I see it, giving some change or a dollar here or there is a small price to pay to placate someone who could turn violent. I actually make a point of putting a couple of bucks in my pocket when I'm planning to go out: I want to avoid having to stop and fish out my wallet (never a good idea) should I choose to give money to a panhandler.

Not surprisingly, I take a lot of heat for this advice. To reward any form of extortion strikes most people as wrong, plain and simple. But keep in mind, I don't pay off that aggressive panhandler out of fear. I know I can physically defend myself if I need to (and by the time you finish reading this book, so will you). But in the interest of safety, I just choose not to. You, too, have that same power of choice. You can pay off a potential troublemaker as I do, or you can turn down his request, keep on walking, or respond with verbal self-defense (as in "Back off!"). Either way, the decision is always yours.

Comments, Catcalls and "Compliments"

Whether you're a man or a woman, it can be nice to be admired; almost everyone enjoys a well-intentioned compliment now and then. If you're on the street and some guy calls out "lookin' good," you may be flattered. Unfortunately, not all comments are so benign. They're typically more insulting and leave a woman feeling not flattered, but verbally harassed.

In my opinion, the difference between flattery and harassment is that one is respectful, the other isn't. And sometimes it's hard for men to understand the difference. I didn't fully understand it myself until I found myself in a situation where the tables were turned. I was addressing a large group of women on the subject of rape. As I finished reminding them, "A rapist can look like anyone, even someone like me," a woman called out, "I wouldn't mind *that!*" Other women joined in with similar comments and jokes. I laughed it off, but inside I felt embarrassed, frustrated, really powerless. I was there in a professional capacity, but suddenly my message was being overlooked. I got a glimpse of what many women have to endure.

I wish all men could become similarly enlightened. Someday I'd like to create a bumper sticker that could hit men right between the eyes:

> *"ATTENTION ALL MALES: Saying 'Nice ass, baby!' to a woman walking down the street isn't flattering, it's OFFENSIVE! If you don't believe me, just ask your wife, mother, sister, or daughter!"*

Granted, some men indulge in verbal harassment "just for fun," truly oblivious to the fact that their listeners find it annoying, embarrassing, or intimidating. So is it right to describe them as "harassers"? One of my students asked this very question. So I asked her, "How do you respond to those kinds of comments?" She replied that she usually just smiles and keeps on walking. Admittedly, she doesn't really feel like smiling; it doesn't make her happy. But her rationale is, "Whatever I do won't make them stop, so why make a fuss?" Well, this kind of response only encourages men to continue acting that way. If you're the object of unwelcome attention, don't "grin and bear it." Don't give men an excuse to continue believing that it's harmless, or even welcomed, behavior.

Not all harassers aim to flatter you, of course; more often, they want to strip you of your power by treating you like an object. Just the fact that you're a woman can be reason enough. By degrading you, they feel more masculine, powerful, and domineering. Interestingly, some of my female students report that they receive more harassment when they're dressed in business attire than when they're casually dressed. This doesn't surprise me. Wearing a suit, these women convey a power and authority that some men find threatening and feel compelled to challenge. But if men use verbal harassment for many reasons, the only thing that matters is how *you* feel about it. If a man's behavior makes you feel uncomfortable or angry, then his behavior is unacceptable, period.

Men in Groups: The "Pack" Mentality

You know what I mean: you're walking past a group of men and become the target for their catcalls, whistles, or comments.

Construction workers have a reputation (often undeserved) for this kind of harassment, but it isn't confined to any particular group. Put men together, and it can often bring out the worst in them. I've seen doctors, lawyers, and stockbrokers harassing women at the health club, on the golf course, and at the office.

Most look on it as a game, a form of male bonding learned at a young age. I know this from personal experience, though it pains me to admit it. When I was in college, harassing women was a virtual rite of passage. During the annual sorority "rush," when incoming female freshmen visited campus sororities, fraternity members would sit on the roof of their frat house, drink beer, and harass female students as they visited the sorority house across the street. That harassment took the form of everything from vulgarities to obscene gestures. Although I never joined in with their harassment, I did nothing to discourage it, either. By aligning myself with my fraternity brothers and remaining part of the group, I effectively sanctioned and even encouraged their actions. Some men grow out of this kind of behavior; unfortunately, others don't. Even so-called mature men can act like animals when in a group.

So how should you respond to verbal harassers? One school of opinion suggests that you insult their manhood. Give as good as you get, so to speak. I strongly disagree. Although this response can be equated with a certain degree of payback, it usually makes things worse. It's difficult for a man to back down when his manhood is insulted, especially when it's done in front of others. So if you're compelled to speak to your harasser, my advice is: leave him an out. Without threatening or challenging him, and without breaking your stride, you can use phrases like "Grow up," or "Get lost." They convey an equally powerful message: Your harassment isn't working!

There are times, of course, when it can just plain *feel* good to tell off a verbal harasser. If you've really had it up to here and want to insult him back, that's your prerogative. Just be advised that you use insults, profanity, and humiliation at your own risk: while they may cow some aggressors, they may challenge others and escalate verbal harassment into actual physical assault. I know one woman who was walking down the street when a man made an obscene gesture in her direction. When she cursed him out with every expletive in her vocabulary, he came after her, yelling

"What did you call me?!" Then, before she could react, he shoved her to the pavement.

There's yet another school of thought that suggests women should try to educate or enlighten their harassers, as in, "Listen, fella: I'm a person, not an object!" If you want to try this tactic, fine; as always, the choice is yours. And it might just work in certain situations. Maybe you're at the office and a group of male workers is giving you a hard time. Ideally, you'd be better off waiting until later and confronting each man individually. Divide and conquer, as the saying goes. But even as a group, these men may listen to your expressions of indignation or requests for sensitivity because they know you, however superficially.

When dealing with group harassers who are strangers, however (and especially on the street), I think any form of confrontation is futile. They usually jeer at women to get a reaction, and confronting them only confirms that they've gotten to you at some level. So does quickening your step, ducking your head, or averting your eyes. This kind of body language only gives them what they want; it makes them feel more powerful. Therefore, my advice is to ignore them.

You may be thinking, "Wait a minute. I've already tried that. I've turned a blind eye and deaf ear and still felt humiliated by the experience." That's probably because you did it feeling you had no other choice. But keep in mind, there are two ways to ignore someone. On the outside, they may both look the same, but while one is rooted in helplessness, the other is rooted in strength. The difference lies within you. Ignoring an harasser *is* a choice, and anytime you exercise your right to choose, you exercise your power. You act from a place of strength.

It all comes down to attitude. Change your attitude towards a situation and you change the situation itself. Imagine, for example, that you're approaching a group of half a dozen men. They're starting to look you up and down, and chances are you're not going to get past them unscathed. "Oh God," you're thinking, "here it comes." You're in a safe neighborhood, you're surrounded by other pedestrians, and you don't feel your safety is in question. So why do you dread what's coming? Because it's six against one, and it's a fact of human nature that superior numbers are intimidating.

Now, let's say that you're out with a group of *women*. As you pass by some guy, he calls out lewd remarks. Are you intimidated? Humiliated? Of course not: you outnumber the jerk, and the confidence you derive from your companions feeds itself. Because your attitude is completely different, you're more likely to burst out laughing, or simply ignore him. Either way, you feel the power is on your side. The two situations I've described are really not that different; in neither case was your safety ever threatened. But the first situation was stressful, the other insignificant. The only difference was psychological.

You can use this type of visualization to help you cope with street harassment. As you walk past that group of men, imagine that you're with a group of women. Or, as an alternative, imagine that you're 10 feet tall, towering over your harassers.

Be assured, group harassers are most deflated, most unrewarded, by a woman who refuses to react emotionally. I had an opportunity to see this in practice when I was on a college campus. A group of male students had congregated. As an attractive girl approached, they let loose a fusillade of whistles and personal remarks. Then something wonderful happened: their "victim" stopped, turned, and without so much as blinking, looked them over with the detachment of a scientist examining specimens under a microscope. She then coolly walked away, having decided there was nothing there of interest. In the face of such calm indifference, her hecklers were deprived of *any* satisfaction whatsoever.

The above example leads me to another tip for dealing with verbal harassers: **make eye contact.** Without breaking stride or slowing down, look at your harasser in a way that says, "I see you, I hear you, but you haven't intimidated me." Without glaring or staring, your look can convey awareness, confidence, and inner strength. It can also protect you: you keep the harasser in your line of sight until you're safely away.

The more you practice the indifferent approach, the easier it gets. There's an old expression, "The dogs bark but the caravan travels on." Verbal harassers are a lot like those dogs: they may be annoying, they may be irritating, but when you come right down to it, they do not matter. So let them bark, and travel on.

Verbal Assault

There was a time when I assumed that "Shake it, baby!" or "Nice ass!" were perhaps the worst things women had thrown their way while out in public. I've since learned, however, that they may also be targeted by comments of a far more graphic and offensive nature. For some women, these comments constitute a verbal assault that leaves them feeling violated, degraded, and threatened. So what if this happens to you? Do you let it pass, or "let him have it"?

Once again, it all depends on the situation. If a man says something offensive to you yet keeps on walking, put your ego aside and let him pass. However insulting or infuriating his words may be, chances are that he poses no actual threat. And lest you think I'm advocating one set of rules for women and another for men, I'm not. Male or female, my advice is the same: verbal or physical self-defense is designed to protect your safety. It isn't meant to protect you from every ugly remark or gesture that comes your way.

This is advice that more men ought to follow, by the way. While we rarely have to endure sexually offensive remarks (gay men notwithstanding), men may be the target of racial or religious slurs, to give just two examples. And all too often, men rise to the bait even when their safety is not in question.

Having said this, there is one type of verbal assault that merits an entirely different response. If your harasser *doesn't* keep on walking, he could easily be a potential attacker. As I said earlier, many attackers test a potential victim for signs of weakness. Making offensive remarks is one of the ways they may do this. So if you feel your harasser is testing you in any way, respond assertively. If you don't, you will have failed his test. He may follow you to a more isolated location—your apartment, perhaps, or an underground garage—where you may be physically attacked. This is a very real possibility.

You should always respond assertively if someone tests your boundaries, and that holds true whether you're alone or see other people around. If you're alone, verbal self-defense is usually the way to go. If other people are around, however, you should also aim to "expose" your aggressor. Keep in mind that the harasser who delivers an offensive remark quietly, under his breath, does so for one very simple reason: he doesn't want anyone else to hear him. Your job, therefore, is to bring attention to his harassment.

> *As Jennifer was waiting for a bus in downtown Atlanta, a man stepped up behind her and whispered, "Hey, bitch." Although other people were nearby, no one but Jennifer heard this man's remark. As she turned to face him, she saw that he was smirking defiantly, waiting to see how she'd react. Jennifer felt that he was testing her.*
>
> *Recalling her empowerment training, Jennifer said loudly and emphatically, "What did you say to me? Did you call me a bitch?" (These were rhetorical questions, by the way: she wasn't looking for an answer.) People turned to stare. Her harasser took one step back, and then another. Finally, he muttered some obscenity and left.*

That man could have responded differently, of course. He might have reacted defensively, or angrily; he might even have tried to strike Jennifer or shove her to the ground. Yet she still did the right thing by putting him in the spotlight and exposing his harassment to others. When you respond assertively, there's always the risk that your harasser will try to escalate the confrontation. But failing to respond assertively can set you up as a target for attack, placing you at even greater risk.

Jennifer used rhetorical questions to good effect. However, I prefer something more direct, such as "Back off, and shut your filthy mouth!" If your harasser utters his obscenity so no one else can hear, repeat it loudly so *everyone* can hear: "How dare you call me a bitch!" Use profanity if you're comfortable with it; the language is up to you. The important thing is to draw attention to the harassment.

The same is true if someone tests your physical boundaries: by fondling or brushing up against you, for example, or by deliberately standing too close. Bring immediate attention to his conduct. "Get your hands off me!" or "Back off, now!" are just two examples of things you can say. You can even use humor. In their inspiring book, *Her Wits About Her: Self-Defense Success Stories by Women,* editors Denise Caignon and Gail Groves recall the woman who was grabbed while riding a crowded subway; "She plucked the hand off her body, raised it over her head, and announced loudly: 'Who does this belong to? I found it on my ass.' Her assailant did his best to melt into the crowd."

If you're uncertain about how to respond in a given situation, ask yourself one question: does this harasser pose an actual threat to my safety? If you think he might, deal with him head on. If he doesn't, let it pass and get on with your life.

Obscene Phone Calls

An obscene caller's whole aim is to elicit an emotional reaction from a woman: embarrassment, shock, fear, sexual arousal, etc. In this respect, he's no different from other verbal harassers, so fight the temptation to argue, tell him off, or bang down the phone. Reacting emotionally only gives him a sense of satisfaction and a feeling of power.

This is one situation where laughter can be the best medicine. I have one friend who deliberately bursts out laughing, then pretends to summon someone else to the phone to "listen to this joker." It's worked every time: the caller hangs up, and never calls back. Another tactic (that doesn't call for play-acting) is to keep a whistle by the phone and blow it right into the receiver. That, too, usually does the trick.

I don't mean to downplay how unsettling an obscene call can be, especially to a woman living alone. It *is* an intrusion, a violation of your personal space. And it's only natural to wonder, "Who is this man? How did he get my number? Where is he calling from? If I anger him, will he try to hurt me?" But the chances are good that he's called your number at random. Most obscene callers are cowards who hide behind their anonymity.

If he calls you by name or indicates any knowledge of you personally, it's an entirely different matter. That kind of caller may represent an actual threat, something I'll be covering in the following segment. In the meantime, never allow your first name to be printed in the phone book or any other directory; you need only provide your first initial. Better yet, get an unlisted number.

Threats of Violence

Most rapists use threats of violence to control their victims, as in "Don't scream or I'll kill you!" or "If you tell anyone about this, I'll come after you." I've met a disquieting number of women, however, who've been threatened with violence in a social or professional context by boyfriends, husbands, co-workers, neighbors, even classmates. The experience can be as devastating to a woman's confidence, self-esteem, and peace of mind as an actual physical attack. Threats are a form of abuse, and you should respond as assertively to them as you would a slap in the face.

Not all threats are made in person. I've known women who were threatened by mail, phone, fax, and computer. One rebuffed a pass made by a co-worker and later found a note stuck to her windshield: "If you report me to your supervisor I'll break your face."

Threats of violence don't need to be carried out to do their damage; if they frighten and intimidate a woman—and render her powerless—they've accomplished their purpose. And any threat, whether obvious or implied, should be taken seriously. I recall the well-publicized attack on model Marla Hanson in 1986. Soon after moving to New York City, she became involved in a dispute with her former landlord over a security deposit. This landlord made veiled threats, then soon afterward arranged for two men to slash Hanson's face with a razor blade.

Don't tolerate any, I repeat, *any* threat of violence. Even if the threat comes from your boyfriend or co-worker, don't dismiss, ignore, or downplay it; take action against anyone who threatens you. Only by taking action will you empower yourself and summon the inner strength your aggressor is so intent on destroying.

Earlier, I encouraged you to try and confront harassers yourself before eliciting outside help. But if someone threatens you with physical harm, forget about confronting them directly! This is no time for false heroics. Instead, get to safety as soon as possible, then respond with other forms of action.

Document the Threat

Documentation is extremely important when it comes to threats of violence. Document threats in writing, word for word, and whenever possible, retain any record of them, such as notes, letters, faxes, answering machine messages, and voice mail recordings. When one of my students received threats from a neighbor, she began carrying a concealed, pocket-sized tape recorder. She got some more of his threats on tape, then took her evidence to the police. It helped convince them that her claim was serious; they visited her neighbor the next day and he never threatened her again.

Report the Threat

If you're threatened at work, immediately report the incident to company security, the personnel department, and upper management. (And remember to put it in writing.) Whether the threat comes from a co-worker or outside "guest," your company has a legal responsibility to provide a safe workplace for its employees. If you're threatened on campus or at school, report it to the dean or principal. Demand that immediate action be taken against your aggressor.

That advice may strike you as simple common sense, but you'd be amazed how often it's ignored. For some people, an appeal to higher authorities seems an admission of cowardice or weakness, an adult version of tattling to the teacher. And no one wants to be branded a whistle-blower or a rat. Dismiss this mind-set with the contempt it deserves! As with any form of harassment, draw attention to the person who has threatened you.

If you're threatened outside a controlled environment (school, workplace, etc.), notify your local police department. Don't believe for a minute that this won't do any good. Let the police know that you take the threat seriously and insist that they do the same. Your complaint will be officially filed, and while your aggressor is unlikely to be charged or arrested, you can and should request that officers be sent to speak with him. This may be all it takes to end his threats; most individuals are intimidated by a visit from the police.

With the help of an attorney, you can also draft a letter to your aggressor threatening legal action. People have been sued in civil court for making threats of violence.

Exercise Caution

Although law enforcement and the courts are valuable resources, there's no substitute for taking responsibility for your own safety. And the first step toward assuming that responsibility is—once again—laying your ego and pride aside.

> *While hurrying to work one morning, Barbara inadvertently drove right through a stop sign, narrowly avoiding a collision with another car. As she pulled over and rolled down her window to apologize, the other driver exploded from his car. He stormed over, berating Barbara with profanities. Then he stuck his face into hers, drew back his fist and snarled, "I'd like to punch your goddamn face in!"*

When Barbara described this incident to me many years later, she was still angry at herself for submitting to that man's threat. Looking back, she wished she'd gotten out of her car and yelled something along the lines of, "Don't threaten *me!* I'll have you arrested!" Surely, she reasoned, that would have been a more assertive and courageous response.

Actually, Barbara did the right thing under the circumstances. Apologizing was the safer way to go. Had she defied that man, yes, it might very well have appeased her pride. But it also could have escalated the situation into violence. Ideally, she wouldn't have rolled down her window in the first place, or gotten into any kind of dialogue with that jerk. As soon as Barbara saw him explode from his car, she would have driven away, and fast.

Years ago, I myself had an experience that was not so different from Barbara's. As I headed down the freeway one night, the traffic around me slowed to a crawl. One driver became impatient and attempted to pass me on the right by using the emergency lane; annoyed, I edged my car forward to stop him from doing so.

I left the freeway at the next exit, unaware that this driver was following me. As I stopped at a light, he bolted out of his car and began banging on my window. He went ballistic, screaming, "You son of a bitch, I'm gonna kill you! I'm gonna kill you!" He had something in his hand that may or may not have been a weapon; in the darkness, it was hard to know for sure. When the light changed, I drove away fast. He leapt back in his car and continued to follow me.

By that point, I was truly alarmed. The last thing I wanted to do was lead this guy to my home, so I just kept on driving. For half an hour, this maniac chased me through the streets of Los Angeles until I finally found a police station. Pulling to a stop outside, I "lay" on my horn. No one came out to investigate, but my aggressor finally gave up and drove away.

> *Nancy was living with her 4-year-old daughter in a high-rise building in Chicago. Night after night, a neighbor in the apartment adjoining hers kept playing his stereo at maximum volume. Nancy finally got so fed up, she stormed down the hall, pounded on his door, and threatened to have him evicted. The man said nothing; he simply stared at her. But a few days later, as Nancy and her daughter entered the building's elevator, he stepped inside. Backing her into a corner, he said, "You yell at me again, I'll kill you and your baby."*

When this incident occurred, Nancy's initial reaction was one of outrage. How dare he threaten her! As she told me, "My first temptation was to yell, just try it, jerk!" But this man was a stranger to her, and for all she knew, capable of carrying out his threat. So she took other forms of action. She filed complaints with the police and with her landlord. Just as importantly, she put safety first. She kept her doors locked at all times. She insisted that her daughter not play in the hallways or outside the building. Later, she moved into her mother's house, only moving back to her apartment when her aggressor was finally evicted. Nancy's story illustrates that you do have options if you're threatened. They may not always be fair, convenient, or affordable, but they do exist.

Ideally, of course, Nancy wouldn't have confronted that man as impulsively and aggressively as she did in the first place. Emotion got the better of her. But if she made an understandable mistake, she didn't compound it by confronting or defying him any further. She decided her safety and that of her daughter's was more important, and acted accordingly.

Nancy's story brings up yet another precaution to take if someone threatens you with violence: do anything you can to avoid that person. Unfortunately, movies and television—even the heroes of history—have encouraged us to believe that avoidance equals retreat and retreat equals "cowardice." As a result, many people feel compelled to go toe-to-toe with anyone who threatens them, as in, "I won't let you push me around!" This is a dangerous attitude to have when it comes to threats of violence. As I said earlier, direct confrontation should be avoided at all costs. Responding with other forms of action is the far safer way to go.

6
STRATEGIES

I'm a great believer in the value of knowing physical self-defense; every woman should know how to fight back effectively when harassment or threats cross the line into attempted assault. At the same time, however, it's important to know all your alternatives to fighting. You run the risk of being injured in any physical confrontation, so it makes sense to try non-physical strategies first; they may be all you need in order to get to safety. In other situations, they may also be used to support and enhance physical self-defense techniques.

Your Voice as an Offensive Weapon

With de-escalation, you use your voice to soothe, calm, and placate an aggressor. Yet your voice can also be used as a strong offensive weapon.

Calling, yelling, screaming: they may all sound like the same thing, but they aren't. In any assault situation, *fight the temptation to scream*. It's unlikely to deter your aggressor. It's what he expects, and screaming only telegraphs your fear.

Indiscriminate screaming can also be misinterpreted. I remember being awakened one night by a woman's screams. When I raced outside to investigate, however, my concerns were replaced by irritation: the "victim" was a teenage girl, shrieking in mock indignation as she and her friends engaged in a water-balloon fight. I think most people have had a similar experience. Unfortunately, this kind of screaming is one form of "crying wolf" which lulls the public into ignoring genuine cries for help. Police files are full of witnesses who heard a rape or assault victim's screams but assumed she was only horsing around.

If you're in trouble, the ideal response is not to scream, but to yell. Yell "No!" at the top of your lungs. Hurl your voice at your aggressor. That's yelling! Try it yourself in a safe place where it won't be misconstrued. Practice yelling as loud as you can, and you'll discover how it energizes and empowers you, just as it would in a threatening situation.

You don't yell to summon help but to attract attention, to "make a scene," which is the last thing any aggressor wants. You also yell to startle your aggressor and catch him off guard. Furthermore, you can use your voice quite literally as a weapon: yell right into an aggressor's eardrum and you'll cause him actual physical pain.

You can also call for assistance, but there's a right and a wrong way to go about it. Don't just call out "Help! Help!" This signals to your attacker that you're helpless and frightened. Instead, be specific. If you see other people or think they're within earshot, yell, "Call the police! This man is trying to hurt me!" Make it clear that you're being attacked, and if you think it's necessary, give your location ("I'm in apartment 4-C! I'm being attacked! Call the police!"). And here's an idea if you're indoors and need to call for help: yell "Fire!" Many people are afraid to investigate an assault situation, but are very likely to respond if they think their building is ablaze.

Here's the bottom line, however, about calling or yelling for help: even if others hear or see what's happening to you, don't assume that they will come to your rescue. In most assault situations that simply doesn't happen. People are often too shocked or frightened to intervene: not only strangers, but people you know. Or they just don't want to get involved. Summon assistance when you can, but don't depend on it. Accept the fact that you will probably be on your own.

Using Your Wits: Negotiation, Stalling, and Other Creative Techniques

Using your wits means, quite simply, using your head. Many women have literally talked, cajoled, tricked, negotiated, and outsmarted their way to safety.

Negotiation can be as simple as saying, "I'll give you my wallet if you'll go away," or "I'll do what you want as long as you don't hurt me." You offer a trade-off. An attacker may not honor his end of the bargain, but you can try this when your intuition tells you that he *might*. Negotiation is one way to appease him, if only temporarily.

The need for power is the driving force behind many assaults. Open defiance can threaten an aggressor's need for power; negotiation, on the other hand, may make him feel he still has the upper hand. It allows him to "save face." Negotiation does work in many situations, and you'll lose nothing by trying it.

Stalling is yet another way of using your wits. It can buy you time until safety arrives or you feel the moment is right to take action. Let's say you've just left a restaurant and your friends have stayed behind to pay the check. You're walking to your car when you're suddenly confronted by an aggressor. You know your friends are just a few minutes behind you, so if you can just keep this guy talking, you'll buy the extra minutes you need to avoid a physical confrontation.

I recall the story of one woman who used her wits in a particularly creative way. Parked at a gas station, she was fueling her tank when she saw a man walking towards her holding a gun. Her intuition told her that she needed to act, and act fast. So she pretended that she knew him. She walked forward, smiling, saying, "Hi! You're my brother Steve's friend, aren't you? How are you?" and so on. Her attacker was confused, and caught so completely off guard that he immediately backed off and left.

When I discuss "using your wits," many women are skeptical at first. Surely, they argue, mere words won't discourage an attack. I don't blame them for their skepticism. We seldom hear about women's success stories and close calls because they just don't make the evening news. Even when they do, they're usually presented in a way that obscures the woman's heroism and success. For example, we may read about a man who breaks into a woman's dorm room and tries to rape her. She manages to escape into the hallway, where she activates the fire alarm and overhead sprinklers. The man escapes on foot. But does the headline read, "STUDENT FOILS WOULD-BE RAPIST"? No, it usually reads, "POLICE SEARCH FOR MAN AFTER RAPE ATTEMPT," or "RAPE ATTEMPT ON COLLEGE CAMPUS." And stories like these are usually buried, while assaults that end with the rape or death of the victim make the front pages. This kind of news coverage can lead us to believe that if a woman is confronted by a rapist, then she's going to be raped.

Don't believe it for a minute! I've heard of women who deterred attackers by deliberately urinating or vomiting, as repulsive as either may sound. Other women have told rapists, "I'm HIV positive, so you'd better wear a condom." Still others have feigned insanity. Tactics like these may be all you need to fool or confuse an aggressor. They may create an opportunity (to fight him off, or to escape) or distract him from his purpose. One of my students feigned enthusiasm, saying "Sure, I'd *love* to have sex, my boyfriend's out of town." Her rapist let go of her arm so he could unzip his pants. This gave her an opening and she was able to run to safety.

Some attackers can be distracted by their own greed. Many women have used the promise of hidden money or valuables to lead their attackers to another part of the house; there, they were able to escape or put up a more effective fight. In author Sanford Strong's excellent book, *Strong on Defense,* he offers yet another good piece of advice. If you're attacked while in your car and forced to drive to another location, don't waste time trying to find a police station or catch the notice of a cop or passing motorist. Instead, with your seat belt securely fastened, crash the car! Even a minor accident attracts attention, and if your attacker isn't wearing *his* seat belt, so much the better.

An attacker may also respond to humanizing behavior. Sharing your name, age, religion, marital status, likes, and dislikes may make you less of an object and more of a person in his eyes. It can neutralize some of his aggression. So can showing an "interest" in him as a person. That tactic has worked for many women, and one of my students in particular. Melanie managed to keep her rapist talking—asking him about himself, feigning interest in *his* problems—and literally talked him out of raping her. (This man was later arrested, and convicted of attempted rape.)

Always be aware, however, that no two attackers are alike: the tactic that may deter one may infuriate another. John Douglas is a former FBI "profiler" and an acknowledged expert on serial killers and rapists; in his book *Mindhunter,* he and co-author Mark Olshaker describe one rape that ended in murder. The victim happened to be a prostitute. Perhaps in the hope that it would diffuse the situation, she played along with the rapist, going so far as to fake a couple of orgasms. Rather than placating her attacker, however, this tactic enraged him: he perceived it as an attempt on her part to control the situation, and it confirmed his most hostile feelings that women were whores. That contempt made it easier for him to kill her. As the authors note, "[This case] does point out why it is so difficult to give general advice on what to do in a rape situation. Depending on the personality of the rapist and his motivation for the crime . . . trying to talk your way out of being assaulted may be the best course of action. Or it may make things worse."

That's why using your wits means remaining adaptable, ready to change your strategy in relation to your attacker. It means remaining flexible, ready to try a second, third, even fourth tactic if the first one doesn't work. Sociologist Dr. Pauline Bart from the University of Illinois conducted a study of effective rape avoidance, first published in 1980. She established that the more strategies a woman uses, the more likely she is to escape with minimal injuries. These strategies include calling, yelling, and negotiating, as well as physical resistance.

One final note: pleading and begging for mercy rarely (if ever) get results. It tends to embolden an attacker, and it's just what he expects.

At this point, I'd like to tell you about Christine. Several years before this young woman participated in one of my workshops, she was home asleep when her roommate and date were forced into the house by three teenagers armed with guns. After she was dragged from her bed, Christine and her roommate's date were forced to lie on the kitchen floor while her roommate was taken upstairs and repeatedly raped.

Christine's intuition told her that unless she came up with a plan to get out of the house, she would probably be killed. So she told one of the assailants that she could get him $300 if she was driven to an ATM a few blocks away. Perhaps tempted by the prospect of easy cash, the kid agreed. With a gun in her ribs, Christine drove him to the ATM and made the withdrawal.

Driving back, as Christine stopped at a light, she noticed that her assailant was busy counting the money. That's when she saw her chance. She dashed from the car, calling out at the top of her lungs. Luckily, she caught the attention of an off-duty police officer who arrested the teenager and called in the incident. Patrolmen dispatched to the house arrested the other two teenagers. A year later, after a long and well-publicized trial, all three youths (identified as gang members) were sentenced to prison for 25 years to life.

I share this story with you to illustrate how, with tremendous courage and cleverness, Christine used **negotiation, stalling,** and **calling for help** to save her own life and the lives of her friends.

Running for Safety

Running is a self-defense option, but only in certain circumstances. Run for safety *only when you know you can reach it.* Simply "hoping for the best" can place you in serious danger, and here's why:

- Running can place you at a physical disadvantage. If your attacker catches up with you, you may be too out of breath to fight effectively. By running, you turn your back on an attacker; therefore, you could be tackled from behind, and injured by the fall.
- Because running telegraphs your fear, it can act as a trigger, making your attacker bolder and more aggressive. It can actually initiate an attack because it marks you as "easy prey."

- If you run and your attacker catches up with you, it's now too late to use verbal self-defense. Your command to "Back off!" will be nothing but an empty bluff; he already knows that you're afraid.

The decision of whether to run or not rests on one of the most basic principles of self-defense: **assessing where safety lies.** If you find yourself in any threatening situation, always ask yourself, "Where is safety?" Is it a few steps away, or a hundred yards away? How far is it to your car? To the door of your apartment? To other people? The availability of safety should determine your response. If you know it's within reach, by all means run for it. If you're in doubt, don't take the chance.

Consider your physical condition—and your attacker's—when deciding whether to run. Be realistic about your limitations. Are you overweight, out of shape, or pregnant? How fast could you really run, and how far?

Finally, if you choose to run, get rid of anything that may slow you down. If you're holding a shopping bag or heavy purse, throw it aside. Wearing a long skirt? Hike it up to your waist. Wearing high heels? Kick 'em off and run in your bare feet.

Nonresistance

When I bring up nonresistance to my students, warning bells go off in many of their minds. "Wait a minute," they argue. "Why learn self-defense if you don't intend to use it?" Yet nonresistance can be your best option in certain situations.

- The first and most obvious is if you're being robbed. If he wants your purse, your wedding ring, even your car, give it up! Fighting over possessions is never, ever worth the risk.
- Let's say you're approached by a beggar or transient asking you for money. If your intuition tells you that he might become aggressive if you refuse his request, take the safe road and fork over that dollar. It's a small price to pay for your safety.

- Nonresistance can be used to lull an attacker into a false sense of security. You pretend to be fearful. You tell him, "I'll do whatever you want, just don't hurt me." Then, when he lets his guard down, *you* attack.

- In a rape situation, your intuition might tell you that nonresistance is your best means of survival. Some experts on self-defense insist that women should always fight back; unfortunately, this advice ignores the fact that every situation is different. What's more, it can leave women who choose not to fight feeling as though they have failed or are to blame. This should never be the case; survivors of rape have a hard enough time recovering physically and emotionally without feeling guilt and self-recrimination.

I've met many rape survivors who cannot forgive themselves because they didn't fight back. Yet their intuition told them at the time that nonresistance—or "passive" resistance—was really their best choice. As one woman recalls, "I got the feeling that my rapist wanted me to fight back, that he needed that reaction to turn him on. So I became as limp as a rag doll, and just as emotionless. He actually lost interest and left."

If you believe your rapist may be deterred by verbal or physical resistance, then by all means go for it! If you feel he is homicidal, you have nothing to lose by fighting back with everything you've got. But just remember: your goal is to survive, and there's no rule that says you have to fight back. If your inner voice says, "Don't resist," then don't. The choice is always yours, and making any choice is an exercise of power.

Having said this, there are times when nonresistance is something I *do not* recommend. If an attacker tries to force you to a secondary location, for example, he's doing so for a reason: he wants to isolate you. It goes without saying that if you are attacked in a populated area, you have a better chance of attracting attention and surviving the attack than if you are taken to a remote or completely isolated location. So never go quietly if someone tries to drag you behind a wall or hedge, down an alley, into another room, or (especially) into a car. The same is true if he's trying to handcuff you, or tie you up. In these kinds of situations, I strongly urge you to fight back with everything you've got.

* * *

I'm often asked, "How many women have successfully defended themselves with your physical techniques?" The answer is, relatively few.

Don't get me wrong: those women who have used my physical techniques have done so with great success. But the vast majority have protected themselves using purely verbal techniques. If effective self-defense means knowing all your options, verbal resistance is one of the most valuable.

At the same time, it's important that you do know how to physically defend yourself if verbal resistance fails. Without the physical skills to back it up, verbal resistance is merely an artful form of bluffing. So don't make the mistake—as so many people do—of learning one set of techniques, but not the other.

There's nothing more comforting to me than knowing that if I find myself in a threatening situation where physical resistance is called for, *I can go to that place.* Because I want you to have this same comfort, the following segments will begin preparing you for physical confrontations.

7
PHYSICAL RESISTANCE: AN INTRODUCTION

Misinformation: Common Misconceptions About Women's Self-Defense

You're certainly at risk in an assault situation if you don't know *anything* about self-defense. But you can be just as hampered by the wrong information.

For most of my students, my seminars are their first exposure to professional self-defense training. Yet most of them think they already know "something" about the subject, little tips they've picked up from other people, from movies and television, and so on. Sometimes these tips are helpful. Usually they aren't, and can lull a woman into a false sense of security. Believe me, the wrong information can literally get you killed.

Myth #1: Kicking a man in the groin is your best defense. In fact, you should never attempt to kick a man in the testicles. Unless you've had martial arts training, you're likely to lose your balance, or miss. Or your attacker may grab your foot or calf.

Myth #2: A man can always protect you. The truth is that men can't always protect *themselves,* let alone you, when it comes to violent assault. If you have a choice of walking to your car alone or with a man, by all means ask him to join you; there's always more safety in numbers. But just remember that safety is never guaranteed.

And in some circumstances, the presence of a male "protector" can actually place you at greater risk. Time and again, macho pride and ego have prompted men to stand and fight in situations where nonresistance was called for (as during a robbery), or when running for safety would have been the far smarter way to go.

Myth #3: A woman should "always" try to run. Not true! As I said earlier, running from an attacker only telegraphs your fear. If he catches up with you, it's too late to try assertive verbal techniques; your command to "Back off!" will fall on deaf ears because he already knows that you're afraid. When you run, you also turn your back on your attacker. He may tackle you from behind, and you may be too out of breath to fight back effectively. Therefore, only run for safety when you *know* that you can reach it.

Myth #4: Size and strength matter. In other words, the bigger an attacker is, the more dangerous he is. This is one myth that most people accept as fact.

Anytime you see a bouncer working at a nightclub or bar, he usually stands over six feet tall and weighs over 200 pounds. The reason is obvious: we naturally find this type of figure more intimidating. In fact, size and strength count for almost nothing when it comes to my style of street fighting! A man's eyes, ears, throat, and testicles are vulnerable no matter how big or strong he may be. And he can't make them any less vulnerable by lifting weights or taking steroids.

Myth #5: "If I fight back, I'll only anger him into hurting me." Or to put it another way, "If I *don't* fight back, he'll go easier on me."

Perhaps more than any other, this is the myth that gets women into trouble. It stops them from fighting with 100 percent commitment, or stops them from fighting back at all. The truth is that attackers don't go any "easier" on victims who don't put up a fight. Usually the opposite is true: they exploit their victim's passivity to their advantage. If you fight effectively, however, the person who gets hurt will not be you but your *attacker*. Get close and cause pain, and he won't have the *chance* to get angry.

Myth #6: Long fingernails make good weapons. While long fingernails (real or artificial) may be used to scratch your attacker's face (a feeble diversion at best), they actually make it harder for you to execute nearly all the self-defense techniques I will be teaching you. For example, if you drive your thumb into an attacker's eye, your fingers should simultaneously dig into the side of his temple, and long fingernails will inhibit you from doing so. They also impede your ability to grab and hold on to your attacker's body or clothing which, again, is an essential part of many of my self-defense techniques. Finally, the longer your fingernails are, the more likely they are to break off in a struggle (and we all know how much *that* hurts).

Myth #7: Women are inherently "delicate." It's true that women are often shorter, more petite, and have less upper body strength than men. Yet none of these things make them delicate! Women are equal to any man in the areas that really count: intuition, objectivity, and "smarts." Men and women also share the same natural weapons. And if a woman knows street-fighting techniques, she's more than an equal fighter: she has a definite *advantage* over the average man.

Myth #8: Women don't have the instincts to fight. This myth is one reason why, until recently, women were barred from flying jet fighters in the military. The reasoning went that women weren't suited to combat because they lacked the "killer instinct."

There's an ongoing "nature versus nurture" debate as to whether male aggressiveness is something men are born with, or something they acquire. Whatever your opinion may be, men certainly have a reputation for being the more aggressive sex. But no one can tell me that a woman's desire for self-preservation is any weaker than a man's. The survival instinct lies within each and every one of us; it just needs to be accessed.

Unfortunately, we live in a society where a man's aggressiveness is widely accepted as part of his makeup, and in many situations even actively encouraged. Meanwhile, female aggressiveness continues to be frowned upon and actively discouraged. Ironically, the aggressiveness which many men bring to a fight often gets them into trouble, fueled as it is by ego and pride. By contrast, the aggressiveness that women display in a fight is usually positive, fueled as it is by a desire for self-preservation.

And even if a woman never feels aggressive, that doesn't mean she lacks the instincts to fight. Fighting is a science: nothing more, nothing less, and you can fight offensively, effectively, and with total commitment without ever feeling aggressive. Indeed, a clinical approach to fighting has many advantages over an emotional one, and I've found that women are actually *less* emotional than men when it comes to self-defense. Men tend to bring a lifetime's worth of aggressiveness, posturing, and "macho" pride with them to class. I seem to spend half my time re-educating them to stop viewing fighting as some extension of their masculinity. By contrast, women generally approach fighting with more focus and objectivity; they're more likely to view it as a straightforward means to an end. That's one reason why I much prefer teaching women to men.

And what about that so-called "killer instinct"? Like many women, you may have been conditioned into thinking that you simply don't possess it. Don't believe it for a minute! I've heard countless stories of women who summoned a rage and fury against their attackers which, far from clouding their judgment, enabled them to fight all-out. And time and again, as I teach women how to fight, I see their surprise when they tap into that "feminine warrior" within. They've always believed that women lacked a killer instinct, then—*boom!*—something comes out of them they never knew they had. They always had it, of course, and you have it, too. So dismiss the idea of feminine passivity and recognize it for the myth it really is!

The Human Animal: Instinctive Reactions to Assault

Animals react instinctively if attacked. They don't "think" about it. Years of evolution have taught them their best defenses. The deer knows to flee, the lion to use its teeth and claws, and so on.

Unfortunately, human beings are not so lucky. Our instinctive reactions are usually the worst reactions to assault. Instead of helping us, they're far more likely to get us into trouble.

I'm always amazed at the number of people who shy away from learning self-defense because they don't believe they need to. They actually assume that they'll "know" what to do, as though adrenaline, instinct, and the will to live are all it takes to survive.

It's true that we have basic survival instincts. If someone tried to put your head under water, for example, you'd instinctively struggle for air. But if we all have survival instincts, our fighting instincts have been eroded by years of civilization. Nature hasn't equipped us to fight instinctively because we don't need to fight every day (if ever!).

Don't confuse instinct with intuition. Intuition is a "sixth sense" that can help you make decisions. Instinct, on the other hand, is an *impulsive* reaction. And some instinctive reactions can endanger your very survival. For example, panic is instinctive. Many people die in fires because their fear takes over and they lose their heads. They do things they'd never have done if they'd been thinking calmly. Or they simply freeze. Either way, their panic makes the situation worse.

In *The Dark Romance of Dian Fossey,* a fascinating book about the woman who devoted her life to studying mountain gorillas, author Harold Hayes refers to the necessity of ignoring one's instinctive reactions when dealing with wild animals. With a charging rhino, for example, you're supposed to wait as long as you dare and then leap to the side, hoping his momentum will carry him past you (and *then* you run). With a mountain gorilla, you're supposed to hold your ground. With either animal, following your natural instinct to turn and run will only put you in greater danger.

I remember the first time I picked up a true crime book. It was a sobering experience to read the postmortem report on the male victim, yet viewed objectively, it told me something about our instinctive reactions to attack. In addition to the knife wounds that actually killed him, the victim had lacerations on his hands and arms. These kinds of wounds are so common that forensic pathologists have a name for them. They call them "defense wounds" or "defensive injuries."

Defensive injuries are just that: injuries sustained by victims as they tried to defend themselves. Injuries to the hands and arms (knife cuts, bruises, scratches, broken nails) are among the most common. The reason is obvious. One instinctive reaction to attack is to put up your hands to shield yourself from injury.

Imagine for a moment that someone is about to hit you in the face. You might scream, throw up your hands, duck your head, back away, or close your eyes. If someone grabbed you, you might struggle to break free. These are all instinctive reactions to attack. But *none of them will protect you* in an assault situation.

If you fell into water over your head and didn't know how to swim, your instinctive reaction would be to flail about, and you would eventually drown. That's why it's so important to learn how to swim. It's the same with self-defense. Self-defense training enables you to make deliberate choices instead of instinctive ones.

The Fear Factor

I would be remiss if I didn't touch upon fear and its role in the self-defense equation. Fear is generally learned, or "programmed." It holds us back from achieving many things, big and small, in our daily lives. Whether it's a fear of failure, success, growth, change, loss, security, vulnerability, or love, fear is one of life's greatest roadblocks.

Attackers use our fear to their advantage. They know that the more fearful their victim is, the less likely she is to resist. The rapist uses the threat of physical violence or death to terrorize a woman into submission. The sexual harasser exploits a woman's fear of consequences (embarrassment, ridicule, even a lost job or promotion) in order to control her.

You may be thinking, "If I just learn enough about self-defense, I won't be afraid." But that kind of thinking will only get you into trouble. No amount of self-defense training will stop you from being afraid during an assault—nor should it. You have every reason to be afraid: you're facing a very real threat! Quite frankly, anyone who isn't afraid in an assault situation is naive about its risks.

In their training, police officers, soldiers, and other professionals are taught that in threatening situations, they should expect to feel afraid. Only by anticipating fear can they learn to move past it and take action. After a plane crash in the Midwest many years ago, some of the survivors recalled that even as the plane was going down, the flight attendants continued moving up and down the aisle, checking that seat belts were fastened and urging everyone to stay calm. Were those flight attendants any less terrified than the passengers? I doubt it. Did they have any less reason to be afraid? Absolutely not. The difference was that they had been trained to move beyond their fear and focus on their jobs.

I've talked to many women who responded courageously during an assault and every single one of them was afraid. However, they managed to channel their fear into action. Remember: courage is not the absence of fear, but the ability to overcome it. And a certain amount of fear can actually help you in an assault situation. It starts your adrenaline pumping, galvanizes you, and mobilizes you to take action. It can fuel an anger, a primitive rage that, rather than clouding your judgment, can be forcefully channeled against your attacker. I call this "healthy" fear.

"Unhealthy" fear has just the opposite effect. It overwhelms us; it paralyzes us. This deer-in-the-headlights reaction is precisely what so many of us dread. The most common fear that my students express when discussing assault is that they will simply freeze, that they will be too afraid to do anything at all.

Fear finds its way into our everyday lives as well. Who hasn't been afraid to ask the boss for a raise, or dreaded a showdown with a friend or loved one? You may be afraid of heights or airplane travel. A recent poll showed that the number one fear most people have is not of injury or death, but of public speaking! The inability to get up in front of a group can cost some people promotions, even their jobs. So fear doesn't begin and end with life-threatening situations. There's more than one way to freeze up.

However, as Franklin Roosevelt said, "We have nothing to fear but fear itself." So when I address the "freeze factor," I immediately go to three key words: breathe, visualize, execute.

Breathing is a key element in overcoming fear. Think about the last time you watched the Olympics on television. Before the athletes competed—runners, gymnasts, pole-vaulters, you name it—you saw each one of them take a moment to concentrate on their breathing. Athletes know that proper breathing is essential to top performance.

Deep, rhythmic breathing will help you stay calm, centered, and focused whenever you feel afraid, whether you're in an assault situation or just asking for that raise. Breathing is a semi-voluntary act—we naturally inhale and exhale without having to think about it—but when frightened or taken by surprise, people often hyperventilate or forget to breathe. Deep breathing will actually help to calm you. That's why it's important to focus on your breathing, to consciously control its rate and depth.

Because involuntary breaths are very shallow, try this simple exercise. Inhale deeply, not only with your lungs but with your diaphragm. (Your belly should push out as you inhale.) Hold that breath for a moment, then exhale. Continue to breathe like this for a couple of minutes. Focus all your attention on the depth and rhythm of each breath. As you do so, your heart rate will begin to slow, your blood pressure will lower, and you'll begin to relax. Whenever you feel anxious, nervous, uneasy, or frightened, try to breathe in this fashion. You'll notice a difference immediately.

In an assault situation, you obviously won't have the two or three minutes it takes to do this exercise. You *do* have time, however, to take a deep breath and let go of any fear, anxiety, and/or self-doubt you might have. As you exhale, "push" those obstacles out of the way; see them disappear.

Visualization is another key element in overcoming fear. I always ask my students to visualize success prior to taking on any challenge. Again, athletes use visualization all the time. The baseball pitcher visualizes himself delivering the ball across home plate; the diver visualizes herself executing a perfect dive. Use visualization whenever you're afraid. Visualize yourself standing up to that friend you plan to confront. "See" yourself hurting an attacker and fighting him off. Never, ever, visualize yourself as a failure or as a victim. Instead, see yourself as a strong, capable, and competent woman, able to meet any challenge.

Execution simply means taking action. Once your breathing is under control and you've visualized yourself handling the situation, go for it. Take that step off the diving board. Open the door to your boss's office. Fight back against your attacker. The first time you face your fear and take action is always the hardest. But the more times you do it, the easier it gets.

Mental Preparation

Imagine for a moment that a school is on fire. For the children inside, being in a burning building is a completely unfamiliar situation. Yet, because they've all practiced fire drills, they *are* familiar with how they should respond. They feel reassured as they get into line, walk slowly and calmly down the hall, and out the nearest exit door because they've done all of these things before.

You can't prepare for a rape or assault situation in quite the same way as you would for a fire. But through mental preparation, you can rehearse your own response. By picturing assault situations and rehearsing your response, you gradually replace the unfamiliar with the familiar. In an actual emergency, you're less likely to be overwhelmed and paralyzed by fear because you have been to that "place" before.

It's only human nature to be afraid of the new, the strange, the unfamiliar. Let's say you were walking down the street and an alien spaceship landed in front of you. Would you know immediately what to do? Probably not: nothing has prepared you for such an event!

Rape and assault can be every bit as unfamiliar as an alien attack, and that's no joke. Few of us have experienced violence before, so it's outside our entire frame of reference. Violence leaves many people paralyzed by fear because it's a completely new phenomenon. Unless you've experienced something in the past, you need time to think about how you should respond to it.

Unfortunately, time is something you may not have in a crisis. Although some situations give you a few precious seconds to plan your response, many do not. I had one student who awoke to find an intruder in her bedroom, his knife pressed hard against her throat. Another was jogging through the park on a nice sunny day with other people around when a rapist suddenly dragged her into the bushes and shoved her down a slope. Attacks can happen this suddenly. They may occur with lightning speed, taking anyone by surprise. Yet, it's never too late to act. There's always *something* you can do. And the more you rehearse your actions ahead of time, the more quickly you'll respond in a crisis.

"Mental rehearsal" is as simple as it sounds. First, picture yourself being attacked. Make your visualization as detailed as possible. For example, what does your attacker look like? How does he attack you? Does he tackle you from behind? Grab your throat? Pin you to the ground?

Now, visualize your response. Do you yell? Call for assistance? How do you fight back? If he hurts you, what then? Will you risk injury—a twisted ankle, scrapes and bruises, even a knife wound—to fight your way to safety?

Don't be surprised if these visualizations make you feel uncomfortable. The very thought of being raped, injured, or killed is so frightening that most people push it from their minds. Fear is the number one reason people avoid learning or even discussing self-defense, and confronting that fear is rarely easy; it's usually downright unsettling. As one woman told me, "When you started talking about the ways I could be attacked, I had an emotional reaction. My heart began racing, my mouth went dry. I even had trouble breathing. Just hearing about rape and assault made me feel afraid." Other students have reported feeling nervous or exhausted. As you read this book, you yourself may be experiencing some of these reactions. Good! You've taken the first step into unfamiliar territory. You've begun to stretch your "comfort zone," and that's the only way you can familiarize yourself with the unknown.

Here's one piece of good news: when I have women role-play assault situations with me, they usually experience more fear watching others take their turn. When it's their turn to fight, they become so focused and determined, they forget to be afraid! The language, shouting, and threats I use to intimidate them usually have very little effect.

By reading this book, you've already demonstrated a willingness to face your fear. That places you ahead of the pack. Most people never prepare for an assault. They hope it won't happen to them or pray that if it does, their reflexes will tell them what to do. There's no substitute for mental preparation, however. It replaces hopes and prayers with readiness.

Finally, mental rehearsal has yet another benefit: it can serve as a "refresher course" for your personal empowerment training.

When my students complete a workshop, the knowledge they've acquired is still fresh in their minds. The same will be true for you once you finish reading this book. But how much will you remember in a year, or in five years? After all that time, will you remember everything you learned? The answer will be "yes" if you continue to visualize confrontations and assault scenarios—and your responses to them—on a regular basis.

Because mental rehearsal helps you to stay current, it will help you contend with the pessimism and nay-saying of others that will continue to come your way. If you've ever been told (and I know you have!) that you couldn't defend yourself from a determined attacker, *don't believe it for a minute!* Chances are that this negative message came from a man, and that really says it all. Many men are reluctant to believe that a woman can protect and defend herself without a man's assistance. After all, aren't women "the weaker sex"? Isn't a woman's safety a man's responsibility? Before you criticize us too harshly for this, bear one thing in mind: it's the message that many of us have been given since childhood.

Listen carefully. By the time you finish reading this book, you will know more about personal safety and self-defense than 99 percent of the male population. And that's a fact!

Making the Choice to Fight

My experience in self-defense has convinced me that certain steps must be taken before you choose to use physical resistance. And the first and most important step is **determining what to fight for.** Too often, people choose to fight for the wrong reasons.

Anytime I ask a group of women, "How many of you would fight for your wedding ring?", a surprising number of them raise their hands. Yet every police officer in the country shares my opinion that fighting a thief over a wallet, purse, watch, jewelry, or car is utterly foolish. Those items are replaceable; you aren't. It's just not worth the risk. Self-defense is designed to defend you, a human being, not material possessions. So choose your battles carefully.

During one of my visits to New York City, the local papers and TV news carried the story of a couple attacked outside their brownstone. A mugger tried to grab the woman's purse. When her husband struggled with him, the mugger shot him dead. The media portrayed this story as "MAN DIES TRYING TO PROTECT WIFE," but they had it all wrong. He died trying to protect her *purse.*

Several years before taking my course, one of my Denver students was attacked. A thug approached Linda at a bus station and demanded that she hand over her gold necklace. He was a threatening-looking character, but Linda's initial reaction was anger: "Who the hell does this guy think he is?" So she refused to give up her jewelry. When Linda continued to refuse, the mugger grabbed the necklace and dragged her across the pavement until the necklace broke away. He ended up with a broken yet still valuable piece of jewelry. She ended up with severe abrasions on her neck, a twisted ankle, and deep scrapes along her knees and hands.

In retrospect, Linda realized that she might have avoided these injuries if she'd simply compiled with the mugger's demands. Her experience illustrates why you should never let emotions or material possessions take precedence over your personal safety. She learned that lesson the hard way. I hope you don't have to.

The second step when weighing the pros and cons of fighting is **setting your pride and ego aside.** I've had the opportunity to visit many martial arts schools, and have frequently encountered ones where the students had a perceptibly arrogant attitude. They exude a bravado, a certain swagger, which they probably picked up from their instructors. Yet theirs is precisely the wrong attitude to have when it comes to self-defense. The best instructors teach their students not to be arrogant, but humble. Everyone needs a certain degree of humility. The best martial artists have it; they never go looking for a fight. The concept of "walking away" is one of the most valuable lessons I've learned from my study of Kung Fu San Soo. I know I can walk away from a situation and still retain my dignity.

In 1996, I was using a pay phone in downtown Houston when I saw a hostile-looking man heading right towards me. Seconds later, he shoved me so hard I very nearly lost my balance, then he kept on walking! Was I angry? Was I tempted to go after him?

You'd better believe it! Fortunately, objectivity prevailed: I realized that while he was being deliberately provocative, my safety was not in jeopardy. So the smart thing to do was to let him keep walking, and get on with my life.

When making the choice to fight, always ask yourself, are you determined to fight just on principle? Are you so outraged at your aggressor that you feel you should teach him a lesson? These should never be reasons to fight. Your unchecked ego and pride can be dangerous, and will only make things worse. As I've said before, men fall into this trap all the time. Their pride often gets the better of them because they confuse pride with self-respect. We've all heard of men injured or even killed because they didn't know when to back down.

The third step before making the choice to fight is to **assess the situation.** Take notice of everything around you. What's your quickest route to safety? If you ran for it, could you reach it? Are there other people nearby who might assist you, or are you really on your own (is fighting your *only* choice?). Can you see your attacker's hands? Is he holding a weapon? Observe your surroundings and your attacker objectively. This will tell you which course of action best serves your primary goal: getting to safety as quickly as possible.

Making note of your attacker's appearance has yet another benefit. When you report your assault to the police, there's a better chance your attacker will be apprehended if you can supply accurate details of his height, weight, age, ethnicity, clothing, and identifiable markings.

The fourth step is to **listen to your intuition.** As I've said before, your intuition is a powerful tool. Listen to it, and trust it. Allow your inner voice to guide you. If your intuition tells you, "If I fight this guy, he's going to kill me," you're probably right. The same is true if your intuition tells you, "I'd better fight or he's really going to hurt me." Every situation is different, and you should choose to fight only when your inner voice, your "guiding light," tells you to do so. Follow this advice, and you have a much better chance of surviving an attack.

Keep in mind that your intuition is sensitive to the ebbs and flows of a situation. Although it might initially warn you against fighting back, *this could change.* In many assaults, the victim sees an opportunity open up that wasn't there at first, so allow yourself the flexibility to change direction at any time.

Finally, **remember your alternatives** to fighting. Physical resistance always carries some risk, and you should avoid it whenever you can. Knowing alternative strategies like de-escalation, calling and yelling, verbal self-defense, and running to safety will enable you to make an informed and thoughtful choice when deciding whether or not to fight.

Now, after emphasizing the importance of knowing all these options, I must tell you that all my years of studying assault prevention have taught me one very important lesson. By and large, those individuals who choose to fight when they have no other option stand the best chance of stopping an attack and reaching safety. Physical resistance is a valuable option in many situations. Just keep in mind that the decision to use it is always yours.

Legal considerations

"How far can I go to defend myself?" is a question I am asked fairly often, yet the legal aspects of self-defense aren't something I deliberately address in my programs. If someone tries to attack you, I think the legality of your response should be the furthest thing from your mind. Convincing women that they can fight off an attacker who is bigger and stronger than they are is difficult enough without bringing legal considerations into play. So my advice usually is, do what you have to do to ensure your safety and the safety of your loved ones, and worry about the law later. To paraphrase a popular sentiment, better to be walked out in handcuffs than carried out under a sheet.

Another reason I don't dwell on the legal aspects of self-defense is that all my assault prevention techniques are designed to be used for one reason and one reason only: protection. Not for revenge, not for retaliation, but for protection. I don't train women to be aggressors. In fact, I believe that the more training a woman has, the less likely she is to use physical self-defense at all.

Having said this, however, the fact remains that you are ultimately responsible for your own actions, so you should understand which actions are legal and which are not when it comes to personal protection.

Though they vary from state to state, most laws pertaining to self-defense grant you the right to use "reasonable force" to defend yourself. This is generally defined as doing what a "reasonable" person would do under the circumstances. You can use as much force as the other person uses (or seems intent on using) *but not more*. In other words, if someone tries to steal your purse, you can't pull out a gun and shoot him; that would constitute unreasonable force. And while revenge may be sweet, that doesn't mean it's legal. If you defend yourself from a rapist, for example, and he takes off running, you're not allowed to get in your car and run him over (however much you might like to). The same is true if you've disabled him with, say, an eye or groin attack: if you have a clear opportunity to escape, you can't stick around to inflict further damage. Under the laws of most states, that too would constitute unreasonable force.

The reasonable force provision is one reason I provide a variety of physical self-defense techniques that range in severity from mild attention-getters, like a kick to the shin, to potentially lethal techniques like a vital-target attack to the throat. If a date becomes overly aggressive, or someone fondles you on the subway, an all-out attack to the eye would constitute unreasonable force; however, a slap to the testicles would not. Knowing a variety of techniques allows you to inflict a degree of pain and injury appropriate to the situation. It gives you the power of choice. Compare this to the woman who relies on a gun for her protection: her options are reduced to an all-or-nothing choice between shooting to wound, shooting to kill, or doing nothing at all.

You should report any type of assault to the police. Do this promptly, and give them an accurate account of the incident. If you hurt your attacker, tell that to the police. At the same time, you may also want to contact an attorney for legal advice. America has become a litigious society; some attackers have taken their victims to court, charging them with everything from assault to attempted murder.

Learning about the laws in your state that pertain to self-defense is an absolute must if you choose to own a gun. No other weapon has the same lethal potential as a gun, and misconceptions about your rights to use one abound. One of the most common is the "man's home is his castle" idea that you can shoot to kill anyone who enters the sanctity of your home. In reality, whether you have this right or not can depend on where you live. In Connecticut, for example, you cannot kill an intruder (armed or not) if you have an opportunity to escape. In other words, you can't shoot the guy coming through the front door if you're in a position to safely slip out the back door. On the other hand, Colorado passed a law in the late 1980s that allows you to use deadly force against a home intruder whether you have a chance to escape from that intruder or not. This was popularly dubbed the "make my day" defense (. . . and the rumor persists that a lot of bodies have been dragged back into homes in the state of Colorado!).

Essential Principles of Self-Defense

As you may have noticed, "fighting" is the term that I use most often when describing physical resistance. I actually dislike the term "self-defense": it's reactive, while fighting is proactive. And to fight effectively, you *must* go on the offensive.

WARNING: Fighting is not what you see in the movies. That's called acting. For example: a man gets kicked in the groin but continues to fight—acting! A solid knee is driven into a man's ribs as he's bent over, yet he continues to fight—acting! A man is hit across the head with a lead pipe but keeps on coming—acting! Enough said.

There are six essential principles that must be adhered to once you've made the choice to fight. Think of them as six "pillars," each necessary to support your effort. If one of these pillars is missing, your effort will be significantly weakened.

1. Believe in your fight. It makes no difference whether your attacker is a stranger or someone you already know. You have the right to defend yourself. Never forget this. If someone intends to harm you, and you choose to physically resist, you *must* believe in your fight.

Society encourages women to be gentle, nurturing, and caring. Nothing wrong with that; they're fine qualities. Yet these qualities work against you in a fighting situation. It's no use going into a fight feeling guilty that you have to hurt someone. You didn't initiate this conflict, he did. When I see women at my seminars having trouble with this concept, I ask them, "What would you do if someone was attacking your child?" The answer is always the same: they'd go after the attacker with everything they had. Your life is every bit as valuable as those of your children, spouse, and loved ones. Believe that, and believe in your fight.

2. Be committed to your fight. Once you've made the choice to fight, anything less than a complete commitment will put you at a disadvantage. Lack of commitment can manifest itself in many ways. It may stop you from using all your power. It may cause you to start a technique but not finish it. Or it may cause you to back off when your attacker screams in pain.

Take the experience of Alexandra, a 39-year-old physician living in Philadelphia. She found herself in a rape situation where she felt she had to fight. She grabbed her attacker's shoulders with both hands and started to bring her knee up between his legs. She had him just where she wanted him! Then something made her stop. Maybe she was reluctant to hurt the guy, or just afraid to fight. Whatever the reason, her hesitation gave her attacker a momentary advantage. He was able to force her to the ground, where she was brutally raped.

Establish a commitment to your fight now; don't wait until you're confronted with a life-threatening situation. I want you to adopt a mind-set well in advance, a mind-set that will prepare you for survival given any situation. Do it now, and your determination to protect yourself will be greater than your attacker's determination to harm you. If you have doubts about fighting with full commitment, if the idea makes you feel guilty, uncertain, or uneasy, deal with it now, calmly, objectively, and not in the heat of the moment.

3. Fight for your survival. More than any other, this principle is the key to realistic self-defense. As children, most of us were taught to "fight fair." But true fighting is anything but fair, nor should it be. The ultimate goal in any physical attack is not to win but to survive.

Unfortunately, most women get their ideas about fighting from watching *men* fight: in movies, on television, in real life. Generally, men are more likely to use their physicality than women; blame it on machismo, evolution, or just too much testosterone. But most of the so-called fights that men get into are really just contests aimed at establishing their superiority. May the best man win, and so on.

That's one reason why men fight in predictable ways. They fight with their strength, their weight, and their fists. As a boy, I had plenty of opportunities to watch other boys fight. And if one of them bit his opponent or tried to pull his hair, he was invariably branded a sissy. He was accused of "fighting like a girl." Many grown men share this same attitude about fighting. They fight to best their opponent. They disdain so-called dirty fighting (biting, for example, or going for the eyes) because if they have to resort to those tactics, they can't really prove themselves the better fighter. Too bad: those tactics work!

Fighting for your survival is a completely different thing than fighting for supremacy or fighting to win: it means doing anything and everything possible to survive. If you must push your attacker down a flight of stairs, so be it. If a shove through a plate-glass window is called for, you'll do it, no questions asked. You need to be ready to do whatever it takes because effective street fighting isn't just punches, kicks, and karate chops: it's biting, ripping, grabbing, gouging, tearing, shoving, tricking, suckering, and everything else that isn't permitted in a boxing match or karate tournament. Boxing, wrestling, and karate are sports. Street fighting isn't a sport but a realistic means of survival.

Many women react with disgust when I explain street fighting's "anything goes" approach. I can see their distaste as I teach them how to tear off an ear, gouge an eye, or bite into an attacker's windpipe. Part of their reaction is simple squeamishness; more often, they're appalled at the idea of hurting another person to this degree.

When this happens, I remind them that, to a great extent, they've been taught to react this way. Society encourages all of us—but women in particular—to recoil from the very thought of hurting someone else, and I myself am no advocate of violence. But I do believe that I have the right to protect myself by any means necessary. I don't find these techniques grotesque or disgusting in any way. What I do find repulsive is violent crime itself: rape, assault, domestic violence, and murder.

Once you choose to fight, forget about what's gross, disgusting, or repulsive. Adopt an objective attitude. Think survival. Remember that self-defense is not an act of violence, but an act of love: love of yourself. You're fighting to sustain life, not destroy it.

4. Fight "smart." Your brain is your most powerful tool for self-defense. Use it! Many women have survived rape and assault by outsmarting their attacker.

Using your environment is one way of fighting smart. Are you sitting at home as you read this book? Look around. You have many household weapons at your disposal: an umbrella, for example, or a pencil, hairbrush, or magazine. Used properly, all can inflict pain on an attacker.

Distraction, stalling, and negotiating are more examples of fighting smart. So is the use of surprise, as when you feign helplessness just before you attack. And so is positioning. Let's say you're in an assault situation and there's a flight of stairs behind you. Fighting smart means moving around to put the staircase behind your attacker, thereby enabling you to shove him down those stairs. Or let's say that the only exit door is behind your attacker. Fighting smart means moving around so the door (and safety) are behind *you* instead.

Exploiting your attacker's weaknesses is another way of fighting smart. Is he limping? Attack his injured leg! Is he wearing glasses? Knock 'em off his head! *Think* smart and you'll *fight* smart, guaranteed!

5. Cause pain. Pain is what I call "the great equalizer" because it can neutralize your attacker's advantages in size and strength. Most women get into trouble because they are reluctant—or don't know how—to cause real pain. They pound on an attacker's chest, when a man's chest is one of the strongest parts of his body. Or they try to break free by shoving or "muscling" him away, which is an equally bad idea. With rare exceptions, a woman's upper body strength will not match up to a man's. That's not an opinion, but a fact.

Here's another fact. You can get around this physical disadvantage by inflicting serious pain. Everyone feels pain. Even when thresholds of pain differ from person to person, a hot cup of coffee thrown in an attacker's face is going to cause him some discomfort. Get the picture?

Let's say you're grabbed from behind. If you struggle to break free without causing pain to your attacker, you're just wasting precious energy. Fighting smart and causing pain *saves* energy. If you bite his hand, for example, heel-stomp on his foot, or drive a stiff elbow into his ribs, there's a very good chance he'll loosen his grip.

If you doubt the effectiveness of a particular technique, think about that technique being used against you. How would *you* react to one of the techniques I've just described? Would you feel pain? I rest my case.

6. Get to safety as soon as possible. Never lose sight of the fact that this is your ultimate goal. As an instructor once told me, "Don't stick around admiring your handiwork." Seize the first available opportunity to safely get away.

Rules of Engagement

Fighting is a science. I never realized this until I began studying my fighting style. Kung Fu San Soo is a Southern Chinese military fighting system that incorporates every aspect of fighting imaginable: not just sophisticated physical moves (punches, leverages, throws, kicks, etc.), but the study of everything from psychology to physics. Often described as a "total fighting system," it can take a lifetime to truly master.

When it comes to self-defense for the average person, however, I teach only the most practical and efficient fighting techniques and principles. With a minimum of instruction, anyone can master them. I do not and could not teach you Kung Fu San Soo or any martial art with this book. Their depth and scope make that impossible. My goal is to teach you how to survive on the street using basic fighting tools. In my opinion, these basic tools will leave you well-equipped to handle any physical confrontation.

Before we begin, let's run down a short list of do's and don't's as they pertain to fighting and self-defense training.

- DO be prepared for the consequences of protecting and defending yourself. If you choose to resist, verbally and/or physically, certain things may happen. Your attacker may threaten you and push you around. He may slap you, push you to the ground, or tear your clothes. You might be scratched or cut. Yet none of these things really matter. They aren't life-threatening and won't compromise your survival.

  Once you've made the choice to fight, you should also be prepared for the possibility that the other person will be injured or even killed. You can't fight effectively without inflicting some actual pain and injury. And if you're in a situation where it's "you or him," the choice seems obvious.

- DO be aware that there are no guarantees you'll never be a victim of violent crime. Regardless of how much training you have, sometimes things are beyond your control. I have a sixth degree black belt, yet not for a minute do I believe that my training will protect me in every situation. Each and every one of us can be a victim, so the lesson is this: live smart, and avoid assault situations at all cost.

- DO think and fight offensively. Don't just react to an attacker's actions; take the initiative. If you choose to fight, go after him with everything you've got.

- DON'T stop until you know you can get to safety without having to look over your shoulder. There's no such thing as "thinking" you can get to safety; you have to be sure. Once you decide to fight, don't stop until you've finished the job.

- DON'T practice the techniques described in this book on a friend or loved one with full or even half force. These techniques can result in pain, injury, and even death. The only acceptable practice is done in SLOW MOTION.

- DON'T be pulled into a "non-believer's" agenda. There may

be people in your life (especially men) who will be skeptical or feel uncomfortable with the idea that you really can defend yourself. They may try to persuade you that your techniques cannot possibly work, even to the point of physically restraining you and challenging you to "get out of this hold." Don't rise to the bait! You don't have to prove anything to anyone.

● DON'T be surprised if you can't "get out of that hold." Unless you're willing to hurt that person, your techniques simply will not work. They only work when you're committed to your fight and prepared to inflict real pain.

All right. You find yourself in an assault situation. You decide that physical resistance is your best option. You make the choice to fight. What next?

Before I teach you actual fighting techniques, I want you to understand that while no two assault situations are alike, and every attack is different, some basic rules always remain the same. These rules of engagement are essential components of self-defense. Follow them, and you'll have an edge over any aggressor.

1. Stay close. That's right! It may go against your very nature. It's probably the very last thing you want to do. But you must get close and stay close to your attacker once you make the choice to fight.

Many self-defense courses encourage women to put as much distance as they can between themselves and their attacker. I strongly disagree with this advice. The only "safe" distance is that which allows you to run and get to safety. Anything less constitutes a definite liability.

When I first begin to role-play attack scenarios with my female students, many are reluctant to get close to me. Theirs is a natural reaction. We allow our loved ones to get close to us because we know and trust them. If anyone else enters our personal space, however, it represents a violation of our physical boundaries. Yet once my students have experienced the advantages of staying close, I've seen their hesitancy replaced by feelings of safety and control.

There's a very good chance that your attacker will make it easy for you to stay close to him. When a woman is assaulted, her attacker is usually all over her from the beginning. See this as an opportunity. This fool has made a major mistake, so make the most of it.

When you're close to your attacker, you have two vital advantages. First, you're close to "targets of attack." You can put a thumb in his eye, grab his testicles, bite his forearm, and so forth. When it comes to inflicting pain and damage, the closer you are, the better. For example, devastating attacks to the eye (which I will discuss later in depth) include grabbing the back of your attacker's neck and pulling his head towards you. And you can only do that if you're close to him.

Second, staying close provides you with a certain degree of protection. Think about the last time you watched a boxing match on television. At some point in the match, you probably saw one boxer "hug" the other before the referee stepped in to break it up. This hug (known as a clinch) is no display of affection. By becoming a part of his opponent, the boxer protects himself from punches and gains a few moments of what I call "safe rest." Picture yourself grabbing your attacker's body, getting close, and burying your head against his chest. You'll understand why this makes it harder for him to punch or slap you.

2. Grab and hold on. This helps you to stay close to your attacker; just as importantly, it increases your stability and control. It makes it difficult for your attacker to shove or throw you to the ground. Grab on to your attacker's jacket, shirt, arm, waist, or anything else available, then cause pain.

3. "Set" your weight. Stability, balance, and control all come from being "rooted" to the ground when engaged in a physical confrontation. Holding on to your attacker, causing pain, and setting your weight should all happen simultaneously.

Most men carry their weight in their upper body; their chest, shoulders, arms, and back are just naturally more muscular than their legs. If this tends to give them more upper body strength than women, it also makes them top-heavy. Men are less stable on their feet, more vulnerable to shifts in balance. It's really true: the bigger they are, the harder and *easier* they fall.

In contrast, women tend to carry their weight in the hip and thigh area. While this may be the bane of many a woman who tries to diet, it gives you a decided advantage in a fight. Thanks to your physiology, you have more natural balance and stability than men do.

When you grab on to your attacker, set your weight immediately. Set it *down* by placing your feet shoulder-width apart and bending your knees outward ever so slightly. Then exhale. Think "solid," "strong," and "rooted." Do this even if your assailant initiates his attack by grabbing your wrist or arm. The expression "dead weight" comes from the fact that it's hard to move or carry a person who's gone limp, and it's harder still to move even a petite woman if she's rooted to the ground. "Set" weight is harder to move. As with grabbing and holding on, setting your weight makes it more difficult for your attacker to lift you off your feet or shove you to the ground.

4. Breathe. This may sound obvious, but it isn't. As I've said before, people often hyperventilate or forget to breathe when surprised or frightened. You need oxygen to fight effectively, and proper breathing (breathing deeply and evenly) will help you stay solid, strong, relaxed, and focused. It's an important component of fighting. When engaged in a physical confrontation, stay conscious of your breathing. Try to *hear* yourself exhale.

5. Be patient. If you've made the choice to fight, don't assume that you must take action right away. If you see an opportunity, by all means go for it. But remember: there's no rush; *you* are in control. You have the means to defend yourself, and you can wait until you're ready. This can lull an opponent into a false sense of security. And because your attack will take him by surprise, it will be that much more effective.

Six Natural Weapons for Self-Defense

Because of my training, some people assume that, compared to the average man, I'm less likely to be intimidated by the prospect of fighting a woman. In fact, quite the opposite is true. I've developed a healthy respect for the damage women can inflict using nothing more than their natural weapons.

Too often, people rely upon external means of protection. Although guns, knives, stun guns, mace, pepper spray, and other devices have their value, they don't change the fact that *you* must be your own first line of defense. The good news is that everyone has natural weapons, and they don't have to be purchased, registered, licensed, serviced, or monitored. You don't have to remember to carry them. You just have to learn what they are, and how to use them.

Natural Weapon #1: Hands. Your hands can do wonders in a fight, but only when used properly.

The most obvious use of the hands is the classic punch, but making a fist and punching looks easier than it really is. The human hand simply wasn't designed to punch. Throwing a punch improperly can leave you with a broken hand, torn ligaments, or both.

Instead of punching, use your hands to *grab* and *tear,* functions they perform every day. Grabbing and tearing can inflict incredible pain and damage to certain areas of the body. I'll be identifying these areas in later chapters.

Depending on the situation, you can also make a fist and "hammer strike" an aggressor's nose, eye, throat, or bladder.

Natural Weapon #2: Elbows. Have you ever been hit full-force in the ribs with an elbow? I have, and it hurts. The elbow (not just the point, but the forearm and area just above the elbow) can inflict a great deal of pain and damage when delivered to the ribs, throat, sternum, diaphragm, and groin.

You don't need to have strong arms to do this. As you prepare to strike with your elbow, twist (or "torque") at the waist and hips to build up power. Then, as you unwind and your elbow hits its target, it will have the whole force of your body behind it.

Natural Weapon #3: Knees. A woman's legs are by far the strongest part of her body. The power generated from a knee brought up between an attacker's legs is incredible. We're talking hospitalization. When I say "knee," however, I'm not referring just to your kneecap, but to the area right above your knee up to your mid-thigh as well.

Natural Weapon #4: The Head. Many of my students are initially reluctant to hit an attacker with their own head, fearing they might hurt themselves in the process. But your skull is made of solid, dense bone, and whether your attacker is facing you or has grabbed you from behind, you can use the top of your forehead or the back of your head to forcefully strike his nose. Remember, your skull is hard; his nose and face are much more fragile.

Natural Weapon #5: Feet. Use the ball of your foot to deliver kicks to an attacker's ankle, shin, Achilles' tendon, and calf. Drive the heel of your foot down onto his toes or instep.

Natural Weapon #6: Teeth. This natural weapon is a personal favorite of mine. Bites hurt, period, and can be inflicted to virtually any area of an attacker's body. Some bites (to the hand, for example) are used to distract, while others (to the windpipe, for example) inflict more serious damage.

Many women in my classes find the whole idea of biting distasteful. They just hate the idea of getting any part of an attacker's body in their mouth. Or they view biting as an "underhanded" way of fighting. One student admitted that she'd always looked down on biting because, "It's what girls do when they don't know how to fight."

Once again, I must remind you of the importance of being objective. Street survival requires you to know all your options. Biting an attacker is simply one of them, and a very good one at that. It's a highly effective and efficient form of self-defense.

There *is* one thing to consider before biting an attacker. Biting always carries the risk—albeit a very small one—of contracting a disease. HIV, for example, is found in the blood and could be transmitted to you from your attacker. Therefore, let your intuition guide you: if you feel this technique will pose the threat of contracting HIV, use another natural weapon. At the same time, bear in mind that rape by an HIV-infected attacker poses a greater threat to your health than the bite you might use to stop him.

Expect the Unexpected: An Attacker's Reactions to Pain

Time and again, I hear women express the same worry: "If I hurt my attacker, it will only make him angry," or "If I hurt him, he'll only hit me harder," or "If I hurt him, I'll just put myself at risk," and so on. I hear this so often, I'm convinced that it's the most common argument against women's self-defense. The irony is, this fear is seldom based on firsthand experience. Most women have gotten it from movies and the media, or they've heard it from other people, especially from men. So many of my students have had a husband, brother, father, or boyfriend warn them, "Don't fight back, you'll only make things worse."

Does that "warning" contain an element of truth? To answer that question, I'd like you to picture the following situation:

A woman finishes work at her office. It's late, and the building seems deserted. As she waits for an elevator, a man suddenly steps up behind her and begins to fondle her. She turns and forcefully orders him to "Back off!" When he persists in his harassment, she slaps him hard across the face.

In this example, the woman probably *has* made things worse by "fighting" back. There's a good chance her slap will anger her aggressor and escalate the situation into violence. But that's because she didn't inflict any real pain. That slap might have stung, it might have surprised and even humiliated her aggressor, but it didn't really hurt him.

If that woman had responded with a forceful slap to his testicles, however, or a solid kick to his shin, she would have been using pain to create an opportunity: an opportunity to turn and run, or an opportunity to inflict more pain and damage. Her attacker's attention would have been diverted away from her and towards his own pain. He wouldn't have had *time* to get angry.

I want you to be prepared to inflict the kind of pain that gets results. At the same time, I also want you to be prepared for his reactions. Fortunately, these are easy to predict. No two assaults are alike, yet we all share the same, instinctive reactions to pain.

Reaction #1: Your attacker's hands will move *towards his pain.* When someone is hurt, their hands move involuntarily to the place of injury. If you bumped your knee on a coffee table, for example, your hands would reach towards your knee. This hand movement is an involuntary reaction to pain. Use it to help you select your target.

Let's say, for example, that your attacker has grabbed your throat with both hands. You might instinctively reach towards *your* pain and try to pull his hands away, but this rarely gets results. Instead, reach up and twist the skin underneath his arm (near the armpit), or drive your heel down on his foot. His hands will reach towards his pain, thereby loosening the grip on your throat and freeing you from his grasp.

Reaction #2: Your attacker will *recoil from pain.* If you're biting his hand, he'll try to pull it away from your teeth. If you've grabbed him by the testicles, he'll try to step back. And so forth. In order to inflict as much damage as possible with your attacking or "action" hand, you must use your other hand to hold on to his body and pull it towards you. You don't want him pulling free the moment that he feels pain.

Your attacker will also recoil away from the very possibility of injury. If he sees you make a grab towards his testicles, for example, he'll instinctively jump back. That's why it's so important to grab hold of him before you even attempt to inflict pain.

Reaction #3: Your attacker may *scream.* If you're unprepared for this, you may be shocked or surprised into backing off. Anytime you hesitate, however, you give your attacker a chance to recover and get angry. And now he knows that you're prepared to fight, so you've lost the element of surprise. So don't stop until you've finished what you started. Don't stop until you can definitely get to safety.

Anticipate his screams (and shouts, yells, etc.), and understand them: they mean your techniques are working! They mean he's hurt, distracted, and on the defensive. They mean you're *fighting!* Surprisingly, though, there's a good chance you won't be aware of any of your attacker's reactions to pain during a fight.

Allow me to explain. When I simulate an attack with a student and she begins to fight back, I gradually escalate the level of "violence." It can become very intense. If it weren't for my protective padding, I'd suffer serious pain and injury. As we struggle, I try not to give my "victim" too much time to think. I want her to react quickly. And because I do everything I can to simulate an actual attack, when I'm "hurt," I scream at the top of my lungs, recoil in "pain," and try to break free.

At the conclusion of each mock fight, I ask the woman to describe what just happened. The response is usually something like "I don't remember much. I saw you coming towards me, I heard you threaten me. I remember that my heart was beating fast. Then I just concentrated on hurting you." But when I ask, "Did you hear me yelling? Did you feel me struggling to get away from you?", the answer is usually *no!* My intended victim was so focused on getting the job done, she wasn't aware of my reactions.

When you have a plan of attack and you're committed to your mission, you're focused on what *you* need to do. You may hear or feel your attacker react to his pain. Because you expect this, however, you can move past his reactions and concentrate on your ultimate objective: ending the fight so you can get to safety.

The Blindside Technique

In most assaults, an attacker tries to overpower his victim with brute force. Yet as he moves in for the attack, he becomes increasingly vulnerable to counterattack. As soon as he puts his hands on you, or wraps his arms around your waist or hips, his hands are occupied. This allows you to inflict pain and injury with greater speed and accuracy.

With most counterattacks to the head or throat, a blindside hand movement is imperative. It allows you to reach your target without giving your attacker warning. It allows you to take him by surprise. The following exercise will illustrate what I mean:

Sit upright in your chair and keep your eyes focused straight ahead of you. Place your hand in a perpendicular position, an inch from your belly. Now, slowly bring your hand up along your belly, past your chest, chin and nose, until it is directly in front of your eyes.

Chances are, you didn't see your hand until it was moving near your face. Your hand was moving up your blind side. Utilize this type of hand movement when attacking the eyes, ears, or throat. It works whether you're bringing your hand up the front or side of an attacker's body. He cannot stop what he cannot see, and by the time he sees your hand, it's too late.

Keep in mind that a blindside hand movement runs contrary to one of our natural, "animal" instincts. Ever see a cat that's been cornered by a dog? It arches its back; its fur stands straight on end. It tries to look larger than it really is. A baboon will roll its pupils back until his enemy sees nothing but the whites of its eyes. The eagle will spread its wings. The wolf will bare its teeth and growl. The puff adder will literally inflate itself with air. This kind of behavior is used to deter an enemy, and it isn't confined to the animal kingdom. When we are threatened with attack, one of our instinctive reactions is to try to look more threatening. We may glower, curl our lips back to show our teeth, adopt a fighting stance, and (especially) raise our arms in front of us. Yet all this really does is give an attacker "early warning," something you never want to do.

Yet another instinct we have is to raise our hand before we try to punch, slap, or strike someone. Don't do this; it brings your hand up in plain view of your opponent. If he sees your hand, *his* hands will come up to stop yours, and he'll move the target away. You would do the same thing. It's a natural reaction.

I recall doing a role-playing exercise with one student who had had some martial arts training. The moment I came at her, she jumped into a classic fighting stance, her hands held up in a karate-type position. Unfortunately, this stance only telegraphed her intention to fight! Once I saw her hands moving in an aggressive fashion, her "surprise" attack was no longer a surprise.

Surprise is the key. You want to catch your attacker off guard.

He's all over you, he's not expecting a thing, and then *boom,* he's hurt! When planning to attack, never move your hands in a threatening fashion or adopt a fighting stance. In my experience, those kinds of actions do nothing to deter an assailant; they only tip him off to your intentions.

8

GETTING THE JOB DONE

Now it's time to begin your private lessons (without paying my hourly fee!). As we begin to explore the finer points of fighting and physical self-defense, it's essential that you understand the difference between **Attention-Getter** and **Vital Target** techniques.

"Attention-Getter" techniques (AGs) momentarily distract your attacker with pain, surprise, or both. A twist or pinch of the skin, a bite to the hand, a kick to the shin, or a head butt to the nose are all good attention-getters. Generally, AGs are only temporary; they aren't designed to permanently incapacitate, so they can be used not only on a potential rapist but on a sexual harasser, groper, or aggressive date. AGs are most often used to create an opportunity or opening so you can (a) flee to safety, or (b) inflict more serious damage. They are great techniques to use, for example, when you want to break free from a grab or hold.

"Vital Target" techniques (VTs) are used to seriously damage or incapacitate your attacker. They buy far more time than AGs, yet are relatively easy to perform. They allow you to genuinely control a fight.

"Attention-Getters"

The following is a short list of AGs, all of them excellent. Keep in mind that some cause more pain—and therefore buy more time—than others. Assessing the situation will help you decide which AG to use. If you're on a crowded subway car, for example, and a man gropes you from behind, a hard elbow to his ribs may be just enough to make him "back off." During a rape or assault, however, you may need an AG that causes more pain and injury (a head butt, for example, or a bite) to break free from your attacker. You can then run for safety (if you know you can reach it) or attack one of his vital targets.

1. BITES. Bites are great attention-getters. Biting virtually any-where on the body will cause some pain and injury. Although it's preferable to bite your attacker's exposed skin, you can also bite through his clothing.

When it comes to biting, technique and commitment are every-thing. Biting for self-defense purposes means causing more than pain. It means causing damage. Think about biting like a pit bull. Your teeth should break the skin, go deep into the target, and come together.

Some bites can be delivered effectively when neither of your hands is free: biting an attacker's cheek or lip, for example, if he tries to kiss you. However, most bites are effective only when you can pull your target towards you. An attacker will instinctively recoil from the pain of a bite, and unlike those of a pit bull, your jaws will not be strong enough to maintain your grip. Therefore, when biting his pectoral muscle, forearm, or bicep, use your hand or hands to pull the target against your mouth.

2. PINCHES. Pinching or twisting your attacker's skin—espe-cially in sensitive areas like the inner thigh or the underside of his upper arm—are excellent AGs for quick releases. And if hairs get caught in a pinch or twist, so much the better.

3. HEAD BUTTS. As I stated earlier, your skull is *hard*. Use it to head butt an attacker's face. If you're grabbed from behind, you can determine where his face is by listening to his breathing or his voice. Drop your chin slightly, then *wham!*—strike his nose with the back of your skull. If you're facing him, slam the top of your forehead (at the hairline) into his nose. Even if he's taller than you, chances are he'll bend over and lower his face (and nose) to your level, making the target very accessible.

4. KNEES. If you aim for the testicles, and bring a solid knee and thigh up between an attacker's legs, you'll get his attention *and* most likely incapacitate him for a sustained period of time. You can also inflict pain and injury by driving your knee into his ribs, or the inside or outside of his upper thigh.

5. FINGER BREAKS. The small finger or "pinky" is the easiest one to break. This technique works best when you're grabbed around the waist from behind: your attacker has no immediate defense from finger breaks because his hands are wrapped around your waist. Grab his finger and bend it *back* with full force until you hear and feel the break. This should be done without hesitation in one quick, continuous movement.

6. KICKS. Kicks to the ankle, shin, Achilles' tendon, and calf are all effective AGs. (Kicking above the shin *isn't* advised; it may put you off balance.) When you kick, remember to flex your toes up and use the ball of your foot. If you kick with your toes, you could break them. The only exception to this is if you're wearing steel-toed boots, cowboy boots with pointed tips, or similarly sturdy footwear. These kinds of shoes are excellent self-defense weapons, and I encourage women to wear them whenever possible.

7. HEEL-STOMP. This is a good technique to use if you're grabbed from the side or behind. It can inflict serious pain and injury to the fragile bones of your attacker's foot. Simply drive your heel down onto the foot and/or toes.

A word about high heels. The sharp, pointed heel of a high-heeled shoe can inflict real pain if stomped down on an attacker's foot, but in most assault situations high heels only compromise your balance and stability. They make it harder for you to run, or to fight effectively. So kick them off if you can; you're better off fighting in your bare feet.

8. EYE POKES. One of the vital targets I will be discussing later is the eye; it's a primary target for vital-target attacks. However, going after the eye with your fingers or thumb is an extremely effective attention-getter and one of my favorite techniques.

Hold your hand as though you're making the "Boy Scout" oath. Tuck your thumb and last two fingers into your palm. Press your first and second fingers together and point them *out*. Move your hand up your attacker's blind side and jab those two fingers into the eye.

9. EYE SCRAPES. With this technique, you bring your hand up your attacker's blind side, then scrape across his eye with your thumb. (Start from the corner of his eye where it meets the nose, and scrape outward.) This attention-getter can be so devastating, it almost qualifies as a vital-target attack. I recall one night at my studio when some black belt students (male and female) were working out in pairs. One student inadvertently scraped a thumb against her partner's eye. The man let out a loud scream and dropped to the floor in a fetal position, his hands clutched to his eye as he moaned in pain. This was a highly trained martial artist, yet it took nothing more than an eye scrape to drop him to the ground and impair his vision for the next 20 minutes. Just imagine what damage might have been inflicted if that scrape had been intentional.

10. EAR BOX. It doesn't matter how big or strong an attacker is, his ear is still delicate. With proper force, striking or "boxing" an ear can inflict serious pain and even perforate an eardrum. To perform this technique properly, don't raise your arm back and take aim at your attacker's ear; that only telegraphs your intentions. Instead, move your hand up his blind side. When you reach the side of his head, strike the ear full force with the palm of your open hand. If your attacker's hands are occupied (around your waist, for example) and your arms are free, you can strike *both* ears simultaneously.

11. EAR TEAR. The ear tear is an outstanding AG: it's easy to perform, yet inflicts serious pain and damage. As I said before, the ear is delicate, no matter who it belongs to! And as an attacker positions himself to overpower you, he often brings this target right to you.

Move your hand up your attacker's blind side and grab the whole ear. Make a fist around the ear (dig your fingers deep behind it), and rip down towards your hip with full force. Imagine tearing it right off! Although that's unlikely to happen, you will severely tear the back of the ear where it joins the head. Your attacker will instinctively grab his ear and pull back, which only helps you to inflict more pain and injury.

Be prepared to see some blood when you execute this technique (the head area bleeds more than any other area of the body). You will also hear his very loud scream. Ear tears hurt! The pain can last all the way to the hospital, and this type of injury requires surgery to repair.

12: THE GROIN. As I tell my female students, there's no area on a woman's body as comparably sensitive as a man's testicles. Even a slight slap to the testicles will cause enough discomfort for it to be classified as an excellent attention-getter.

To give you an idea of just how delicate the testicles are, stop reading for a moment and slap yourself solidly on the shoulder. The slight pain will not even make you flinch. I can assure you, that same slap to a man's testicles will cause enough pain to make him buckle at the waist and reach for his groin.

Slaps to the groin are painful, but not permanently debilitating. Therefore, they're best suited to situations where your life isn't in danger but you still want to send a man a clear message to "back off." They can be used against a date, for example, if he persists in making unwelcome physical advances, or against a stranger when other people are around:

Elizabeth was in a crowded elevator when a man standing behind her groped her between the legs. She could have responded with verbal self-defense, but decided to use an attention-getter instead. With his body pressed against hers, she knew exactly where he was. So without turning to look at him, Eliza-

beth reached behind her and slapped the man's groin. He grabbed his crotch and actually fell to his knees. (He was also humiliated in front of others.) The doors opened moments later and Elizabeth calmly left the elevator. Her aggressor was still on his knees, moaning in pain.

If your aggressor is behind you, you can also make a fist and use the *padded bottom of that fist* to "hammer strike" back at his groin or lower abdomen.

"Vital-Target" Attacks: The Three Best Targets for Self-Defense

Vital-target (VT) attacks inflict the most pain and damage. They're your very best bet when it comes down to your survival. Although some AG attacks might cause injury, VT attacks leave little doubt that your attacker will be stopped.

Vital-target attacks focus on the **eyes, throat,** and **groin.** Effective self-defense dictates that you go after your attacker's weakest points, and these three areas are his most vulnerable. They're also accessible; when your attacker is all over you, at least one of these areas will be within reach.

1. THE EYE. The eye is my favorite VT area. It's *the* vital target of choice. If you have two free hands, and your survival is in question, go after the eye. Although surrounded by bone, the eye itself is unprotected. It's extremely vulnerable to frontal, full-force attacks with fingers, objects, and especially the thumb. The most devastating self-defense technique of all is literally at your fingertips.

In Richard Preston's riveting best seller *The Hot Zone*—describing an outbreak of the deadly Ebola virus among laboratory monkeys in suburban Washington D.C.—he explained why a 10-pound monkey and a 200-pound man are pretty evenly matched in a fight. A monkey "will grab you by the head, using all four limbs, and then it will wrap its tail around your neck to get a good grip, and it will make slashing attacks all over your face with its teeth, *aiming especially for the eyes."* He goes on to say that "The monkey will be *all over the man.* By the end of the fight, the man may need hundreds of stitches, and could be blinded."

The italics in the previous quotations are my own, to emphasize one obvious fact: by getting close to its "opponent" and targeting the eyes, even a small monkey can inflict serious damage. And what the monkey does instinctively, you can do with a minimum of instruction.

An attack to the eye can inflict serious pain and injury, and possibly permanent damage. Yet the technique itself is very easy to learn. To execute it properly, your movements must be forceful. You also need to be close. If he's trying to hug, kiss, or grope you, so much the better: he's bending forward and bringing the target right to you. Both your hands should be near your chest. Your **action** hand executes the actual attack while your **non-action** hand plays a supporting role.

Use your non-action hand to hook the back of your opponent's neck. Cup the back of his neck with your hand and pull him down (not forward) towards your chest. Keep your elbow tight and close to your body; this enables you to pull his head with greater force. The farther away your elbow is from your body, the less control you have over your attacker. Keep your feet apart: ideally, one foot is slightly closer to your attacker than the other. Give yourself the most stability that you can.

Now breathe deeply, set your weight, and use *all your body weight* to pull him down towards your shoulder. Even when your attacker is bigger or taller than you are, his neck muscles will not be able to match the strength of your body weight. He'll be bent over in an uncomfortable position and his vision will be obstructed. You'll be *pulling him into the attack.* As your action hand moves towards his eye, he won't be able to pull away.

As you hook the back of your attacker's neck, use your action hand to attack the eye itself. To visualize the correct position of the hand, pretend for a moment that you're holding a glass and making a toast. In this position, you'll see that your hand is open yet curved, your thumb extended out, and your fingers pressed together.

Move your action hand up your attacker's blind side and drive your thumb forcefully into the inside corner of the eye (where it meets the nose). Once your thumb is in the eye, use your fingers to grip and squeeze the side of his head. Try to close your hand into a fist. Think of the human skull as a bowling ball: your thumb pushes into the thumb-hole (the eye) while your fingers grip the ball (his skull). With your non-action hand cupping the back of his neck, your thumb deep in his eye socket, and your fingers gripping and digging into the side of his head, your attacker will be locked in. He will be trapped right against your body.

As you drive your thumb into his eye with your action hand, continue to pull his head down towards your chest and the shoulder of your non-action hand. Remember, your action and non-action hand must move simultaneously. Meanwhile, tuck both your elbows in tight and close to your body.

Here's what to expect as you jerk his neck forward and attack the eye. His head and neck will instinctively pull back in a whiplash-type movement. He's going to scream, and he's going to struggle madly to get away from you. Both of his hands will move involuntarily towards his pain as he grabs your hand and tries to pull your thumb out of his eye. He will stagger forward to try and keep his balance. That's why it's important to keep your weight down and solid. Back yourself against a wall, door, or railing if you can for extra support.

Your attacker will have no idea what's happening until it's too late. One second he's fine, the next second he's in horrendous pain. Many people think that this kind of attack will push the eye right out of its socket. While that won't happen, you will severely damage the eye and possibly cause permanent blindness. Don't let that deter you: stay objective when it comes to fighting and self-defense. Remember, you're fighting for your survival.

If you press your thumb into his eye for a good five to ten seconds, that's certainly enough time to inflict serious damage. But if you feel that he's still able to fight, stay with it. Don't release him until you feel he's been immobilized, until you've "knocked the fight right out of him." If he falls to his knees, for example, yet he still seems capable of resistance, drop to one knee and maintain your hold and balance. Don't let go until you know you can get to safety.

As soon as your attacker goes weak and limp, as soon as he

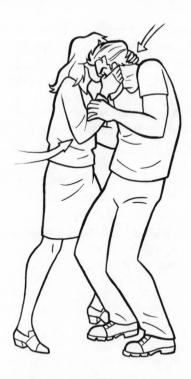

**Vital-Target attack to the
eye (full view)**

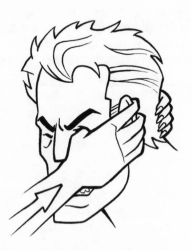

**Vital-Target attack to the
eye (close up)**

begins to sag against you, feel heavy, or collapse to the ground, it probably means that he's on his way out. He may even be losing consciousness or going into shock. (Keep in mind, this *is* a traumatic injury.) *Don't try to hold him up.* Turn his head towards your non-action hand and shove him forcefully to the ground.

It's essential that you turn his head before you shove him. Where the head goes, the body goes. By turning his head, you put him off balance. And remember to *open your action hand* as you shove. If you don't, he may bring you down with him.

Now is as good a time as any to talk about falls and their value in self-defense. Don't underestimate the damage that can be inflicted on your attacker with a forceful push or shove when he's off balance. A twisted ankle or knee, a bruised or fractured hip, torn ligaments in the wrist, a shattered elbow, an injured shoulder or back, and concussion are just a few of the many injuries that can be sustained from a fall.

2. THE THROAT. While attacks to other vital targets inflict both pain and injury, those to the throat can actually result in death. They inhibit your attacker's very ability to breathe.

When you attack the throat, you attack the windpipe. Made of cartilage, the windpipe is a delicate area that can be severely damaged by a strike or grab. Any attack to the throat will be painful and frightening for your attacker. Damaging the windpipe will stop him in his tracks. There are three types of attacks targeted at the throat: the **strike,** the **grab,** and the **bite.**

To **strike** the throat, bring your open hand (curved in the "toast"-like fashion described earlier) up along your attacker's blind side. Slam it into the *front* of his throat. Don't push at the throat; strike it full-force. Keep your hand solid and strong. Hit *through* the throat. Visualize hitting his windpipe out the back of his neck.

The windpipe runs the entire length of his throat, and you can hit it anywhere as long as you hit the *front* of his neck. It doesn't matter if your attacker is a body-builder with an 18-inch neck: he has no muscular protection at the front of the throat.

Striking the throat with your open hand is better than punching it with your fist. If your attacker drops his head, you won't be able to reach his throat with a punch. (This is one reason a boxer is taught to keep his chin down.) With an open hand, *you can't miss*. As long as you're close, your strike will be right on the money. And moving your hand up your attacker's blind side means he won't be able to see or intercept it until it's too late.

Grabbing is the second way to inflict pain and damage to the throat. Grabs are best executed when you have two free hands.

When you grab the throat, don't try to wrap your thumb and fingers around the neck. Chances are that your attacker's neck circumference (and the size of your hand) would prevent you from getting a solid grip. Instead, bring your open hand up your attacker's blind side, grab his throat, and dig your fingers and thumb *into* his voicebox and windpipe as though you're trying to squeeze them into a fist. (Remember: long nails will impede your ability to make a solid fist.) Squeeze with all your strength, and rip outward. Visualize grabbing the windpipe and tearing it out of his neck. The strength of a child is all that is needed to put a large man down with this kind of attack.

The strike and the grab are most effective when you simultaneously use your non-action hand to hook your attacker's neck and pull him towards you. This allows you to inflict damage more forcefully and accurately because it stops him from moving away from your action hand. (And believe me, he will try to move back.) If you have only one hand free, however, just remember that strikes and grabs will still inflict some pain and injury.

When you grab his throat, he'll instinctively try to pry your hand away. *He may eventually succeed.* However, this is not going to be an easy thing for him to do if you dig your fingers into his windpipe, use your other hand to pull him towards you, and stay with him. By the time he pulls your attacking hand away, you will have already inflicted serious damage.

Finally, if you have both hands free, you can also **bite** your attacker's throat. Wrap both your hands behind his neck and pull him tight against you as you simultaneously sink your teeth into his windpipe. Crushing this delicate area with your teeth can be accomplished quickly.

With any attack to the throat, don't expect your attacker to scream. Damaging the windpipe hinders his ability to inhale oxygen; if he can't breathe, he can't scream. His eyes will go wide with surprise and fear. The throat is a very frightening place to be hurt, no matter who you are.

3. THE GROIN. For most women, a man's groin is the first target they think of when it comes to self-defense. And with the proper technique, an attack to the groin *can* literally drop an attacker in his tracks.

Attacks to the groin are aimed not at the penis but at the testicles. A man's testicles are extremely sensitive. Crushing them in your fist or striking them with your knee will cause extreme pain and damage. In real life, men who are attacked in this area are usually finished.

As I said earlier, never attempt to kick a man in the testicles. Too many things could go wrong with a kick: he could grab your foot or leg, you could lose your balance, or you could just plain miss. Instead, I recommend that you attack the groin area with your hand or knee. When using your hand, you have the option of striking or grabbing the groin.

Striking the groin is an excellent technique because you only need one hand to execute it. Striking the groin means using the heel area of your hand, with your fingers pointed down towards the ground. Hit the testicles with your hand *from your hip;* this will give you maximum power and strength. As with other attacks, stay close and strike *through* your target.

Grabbing the groin is another terrific way to stop an attack. It works best when an attacker is wearing loose-fitting pants (dress slacks, sweatpants, shorts), or when he isn't wearing any pants at all. Grab the testicles and crush them in your fist with all your strength. You'll also grab surrounding hair and skin, and that's fine! The idea is to inflict as much pain as possible. If he isn't wearing any pants, tear the testicles as you crush them in your fist. Visualize tearing them right out of his body, pulling your fist towards your hip.

Grabs to the groin work best when you have both hands free. As you use your action hand to attack the testicles, place your non-action hand at your attacker's lower back or buttocks. This gives you leverage and stops him from instinctively moving back.

When you use your knee to attack the groin, grab hold of your attacker's clothing (shirt, jacket) at the chest area, or if he's bare-

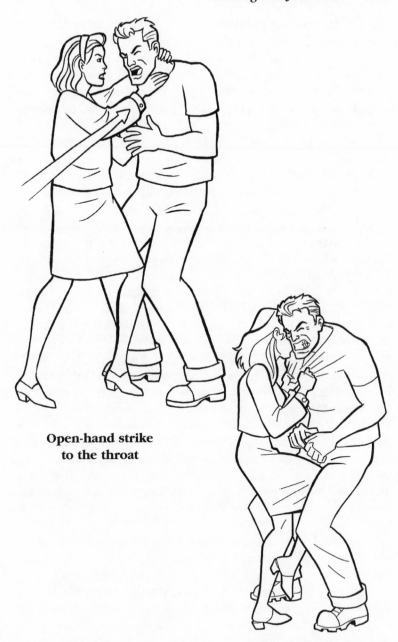

**Open-hand strike
to the throat**

Knee to the groin

chested, by hooking the back of his neck. Stay close, and drive your leg up *forcefully* between his thighs. You want to hit his testicles with the part of your thigh that is just above the knee; this ensures you'll make contact with your target. Remember, your legs are the most powerful part of your body. Use them! *Stay close* to your attacker as you bring your leg up! Any distance between the two of you will allow him to see what you're up to. As with all other attacks, surprise is the key to achieving maximum effectiveness.

When you strike, grab, or knee the testicles, be sure to stand to either side of your attacker, never directly in front of him. Once he's hurt, your assailant will reach for his groin, bending at the waist and dropping his head. If you're standing directly in front of him, you're likely to bump heads. It's also very likely that your attacker will buckle at the knees and begin to drop to the ground. Don't go down with him! If you've immobilized him enough, run for it! If you think he might still hurt you, go after his eye or throat.

Not all attacks take place with both parties standing up. There's always the possibility of an attacker forcing a woman to her knees to perform oral copulation. This is a common attack scenario. Sexual assaults are motivated by a desire for power and control rather than sex; an attacker aims to control, degrade, and humiliate his victim. Forced oral copulation is one of the ways in which he tries to do this.

I need you to see this as yet another opportunity. In many rapes performed by one assailant, fellatio is forced *with no weapon in evidence.* You're in a position, therefore, to strike his testicles, or grab and crush them. You can also bite into his penis. All of these attacks will inflict traumatic injuries and stop this guy in his tracks. Surgery and hospitalization will be required to put him back together.

Your attacker will almost certainly threaten to hurt or even kill you if you try to hurt him while you're on your knees. He wants you to be afraid; in fact, he's banking on it because he knows he's in a vulnerable position. And you may be too afraid to try anything for fear of being punched or strangled. After all, you're on your knees in a "submissive" position, he's standing over you, and he's probably grabbing your head and hair. So it's natural for you to feel helpless.

But stop right there. The person threatening you with bodily harm is standing there with his penis inside your mouth. His pants may be down, which means that his testicles are exposed and within your reach. *Now which one of you is more vulnerable?* The answer is obvious. Make no mistake about it, if you bite into your attacker's penis, or grab and crush his testicles in your fist—or better yet, do both simultaneously—he will have neither the desire or capability of hurting you any further. He will be focused on his own traumatic injuries and pain. So ignore his threats, and take action.

Household Weapons

Say "weapon," and most people think of a knife or a gun. But now that you know about the vulnerable areas of an attacker's body, you can target them with what I call "household weapons." These are everyday objects found in your home, workplace, or car that can be used for self-defense. Accessible, legal, and effective, they can supplement your own natural weapons.

The best household weapons are readily accessible and fit easily in your hand. Pens and pencils, for example, make particularly good household weapons. If you're attacked from the front, bring your pen or pencil up your attacker's blind side and, gripping it as you would a knife, thrust it into his eye, throat, belly, groin, or thigh. If you're attacked from the rear or the side, drive your weapon into his upper thigh, outer thigh, or groin. Believe me, this will cause pain!

A rolled up magazine (the thicker the better) is yet another good household weapon; it can inflict serious pain and injury if thrust into an attacker's eye, throat, or groin. So can a book, umbrella, kitchen utensil, coffee mug, or the handle of a hairbrush. The idea is to use what's available. For example, Donna was surprised by an aggressor at her office. Lacking a conventional weapon, she grabbed a pot of hot coffee and hurled it towards his face. This gave her the few seconds she needed to run into another room, lock the door, and phone for help. Yet another student was cleaning her apartment when the doorbell rang. As she opened the front door, a man forced his way inside. This woman was holding a broom at the time; fortunately, she didn't use it to swat at the intruder, but instead jabbed its blunt end straight into his groin. He was sufficiently disabled for her to shove him back outside, lock the door, and call the police.

As the above examples illustrate, household weapons can be used for both vital-target and attention-getter attacks. Select your target based on the amount of time you need to get to safety. For example, a quick pencil thrust to the belly or bicep is an excellent attention-getter, and may be just enough to do the job.

The real beauty of household weapons is that they are not perceived as a threat. If you face an attacker with a kitchen knife in your hand, he'll view it as a weapon and react accordingly. Face him holding a coffee mug or pen, however, and as far as he's concerned, you're unarmed. If and when you do employ your weapon, therefore, surprise will be on your side. Surprise is crucial, so always keep your weapon low and at your side; this will allow you to attack from any position. And when you do attack, bring your weapon up your assailant's blind side.

I mentioned kitchen knives earlier for a reason: they're usually at the top of the list when I ask students, "If you were attacked in your home, what household weapon would you try to arm yourself with?" Unfortunately, there are several problems associated with using a knife, or for that matter, a pair of scissors or shears. One, your attacker will see it for the weapon it is and be instantly on his guard. Two, knives have very limited value as deterrents; while they may scare off some aggressors, I wouldn't depend on that happening. Three, unless you've been trained to use a knife, you have no more than a fifty-fifty chance of hurting your aggressor. Finally—and most importantly—you run the real risk of losing a knife in a struggle and having it used against *you*.

Many people keep a baseball bat or policeman's baton under the bed to use against an intruder. Like knives, however, bats or batons are perceived as weapons, so forget about making a surprise attack. They also require a certain amount of upper body strength to use effectively. Most women, therefore, are better off using an object which is easy to handle, easy to conceal, and nonthreatening in appearance.

Because attackers look for easy prey, the elderly continue to be among their favorite targets. However, some elderly people carry a cane, and if used properly, a cane can serve as a very effective weapon. Jab the blunt end into his ribs, bladder, or (ideally) his groin. A jab can cause real pain and injury, yet takes surprisingly little strength to execute. A cane can also be used in a "golf-type" swing against the bony parts of your attacker's leg: ankle, shin, or knee.

Remember: it's not the object that counts so much as how you use it. Even the most commonplace or seemingly harmless item becomes an effective weapon when directed towards the vulnerable parts of the human body. Household weapons are often at your fingertips, so use them!

Defenses Against Slaps and Punches

This is one of the most important self-defense skills that you need to learn. Your head is usually the intended target when an attacker tries to slap you with his open hand or punch you with his fist. It's crucial to protect your head because your brain is the "master computer" of all your bodily functions. A solid blow to your head can short-circuit brain activity, knocking you unconscious or leaving you too dizzy or disoriented to fight.

Protecting your head isn't difficult, however. When your attacker is about to punch or slap you (and you'll usually see it coming), the first thing to do is position yourself. The best place to be is either beyond your attacker's reach, or in his face. If you can't get away in time, get close instead, and it will be impossible for him to punch or slap your head with any force. Remember the boxer's clinch or "hug" I referred to earlier? That hug will help protect your head from a serious punch or slap. Simply wrap your arms around your attacker, hug him like there's no tomorrow, and tuck your head into his chest. Become a "part" of him, and don't let go of him until you're ready to attack. Then dig your nails into his back, sink your teeth into his pectoral muscle, slide your hands up to attack his eye, ear, or throat, or drop your hand down to his groin. Get the picture?

The next best defense is to use your arms (not your hands) to shield your head and face. Your attacker may try to strike you with a "haymaker," namely, a forceful blow with his fist. This is the norm for most men. As he begins to wind up for the punch, he'll drop his arm and shoulder back to build up power. Then he'll swing that side of his body towards you.

His body movements give everything away, telegraphing his intention to punch or slap you. The moment you see them, bring both of your arms up to your head and cup the rear of your neck with both hands. Press your forearms flush against your ears with your elbows pointed towards him. If he's grabbed one of your arms, you can still use your other arm to protect your head.

Don't be surprised if his strike hits you in the arm. However, as long as your forearms are held tightly to your ears, your head and face will be protected. However painful a punch or slap to the arm can be, it's a small price to pay to protect your body's "computer center." If your attacker is taller than you (and unarmed), he may try to hit the top of your head with his fist. Don't worry: the top of your skull is solid bone and he's more likely to hurt *himself* in the process.

When we see something heading towards our face, we instinctively duck or drop our head, and avert or close our eyes. Don't do any of these things! Always keep your head up and your eyes focused directly on your attacker. Don't take your eyes off him for a second.

Moving the target. Getting close and becoming a "part" of your attacker. Pressing your forearms against your ears with your elbows pointed out. Now that I've explained these three techniques, it's time to emphasize one very important point: often the very best way to protect yourself from slaps or punches—or indeed any physical strike—is to *go on the offensive.* In Tim Green's book, *The Dark Side of the Game,* chronicling his days as an NFL defensive lineman, he emphasizes that the best way a player can protect himself is by *attacking* with total commitment. Why? Because moving slowly, defensively, or hesitantly gives your opponent time to react and therefore increases your chances of getting hurt. I myself remember one football coach exhorting me to charge down the field like a "freight train out of control." He understood that the sheer momentum of a determined assault can not only carry a player to victory but also protect him in the process.

It's really true: the best defense is a good offense. So if you believe your safety is in jeopardy, take the initiative. You may feign helplessness initially, luring your aggressor into a false sense of security, but I wouldn't always wait for him to make the first move. Attack him before he has a chance to attack you.

Even in the studio, my San Soo workouts are as different as night and day when I think and fight offensively, and when I don't. When I attack, I'm acting rather than reacting. My opponent isn't controlling the fight, I am. When I fight defensively and reactively, however, nothing seems to work: I'm slow, hesitant, off balance, and out of sync. *I'm also more likely to get hurt.* And what applies to San Soo, or the game of football, applies to the serious business of assault prevention. So stay focused, move forward, and go on the offensive.

And whenever possible, carry this mind-set into other areas of your life. A defensive attitude will handicap you not only in assault situations, but in your day-to-day existence. It's all too easy to live reactively, allowing others to dictate your decisions, your actions, your very future. Taking control of your life requires action, not reaction; it means taking the initiative and going on the offensive. Show me a woman who's not afraid to take control of her life, and I'll show you a woman who, with just a little bit of knowledge, can fight her way to safety.

Finding Freedom: Easy Escapes from Grabs, Holds and Chokes

An attacker usually initiates an assault with a grab, hold, or choke to restrain his victim and bring her under his control. However, you may also be grabbed by someone who simply wants to intimidate, manhandle, or threaten you. Whatever the situation, you can free yourself from these temporary restraints by employing some simple yet effective techniques. The key is not to panic. Take your time, take a deep breath, and remember that you are in control.

1. GRABS. Many attacks begin with an aggressor grabbing your wrist or arm. You may be grabbed from any direction: front, side, or rear. I need you to recognize that when your attacker grabs you, he puts himself at a disadvantage: he now has only one free hand with which to hurt you. Advantage: *you.*

Your immediate, natural reaction if someone grabs your wrist or arm may be to pull away. Don't even try this! It's unlikely to work, and you'll expend precious energy fighting against his strength. However, twisting out of a grab is possible. Let's say someone is holding your arm. Bring that arm up and around in a circular motion: in front of your body, around, and down. (Try it.) This forces your aggressor's hand to adjust to the movement of your arm. The weakest part of his grasp is where his thumb and fingers meet around your arm, and a circular motion will expose this weakness. He'll be forced to adjust or loosen his grip, giving you just enough leverage to escape his grasp.

An even better way to free your captured wrist or arm is to close your captured hand into a fist (palm up), then grab that fist with your other hand. Now, forcefully pull your fist back towards your "free" shoulder. Set your weight back and down as you do this and it will be virtually impossible for your attacker to maintain his grip.

The very best way to break free when an aggressor grabs your arm, however, is to forget about your captured arm altogether. Instead, use one of your other natural weapons to *cause pain*. Grab and tear his ear, drive your knee into his testicles, kick him in the shin, or bite him on the cheek. Use any of the other attention-getter or vital-target techniques which I've described. Even if an aggressor grabs your clothing—your collar or sleeve, for example—causing pain is your best way of breaking free. Then you can either run to safety (if you know you can reach it), or go on the attack and inflict more pain and injury.

Remember: an attacker can't protect every area of his body. There's always a target available, and you'll be able to use at least one of your natural weapons. I actually welcome a grab because it means an aggressor's hand or hands are occupied. It puts *him* at a disadvantage.

It's not uncommon for an attacker to grab or pull a woman's hair. Children do this all the time when fighting. I'll never forget seeing two 9-year-olds go at each other while I was working at a summer camp as a teenager. In addition to wildly swinging and kicking, they both tried to grab and pull the other's hair. But when an attacker grabs your hair, he puts himself at an even greater disadvantage than if he grabs your wrist or arm. Why? Because it means that you have *both* hands free with which to fight.

If someone grabs us by the hair, we instinctively try to pull away. Fight the urge to do this; you'll just make the pain worse. Instead, do just the opposite: move in the direction you're being pulled. Get as close as you can to your attacker. This will make it easier on your scalp and make it easier for you to inflict pain. If he's behind you, back up with him. If he's to the front or side, move in that direction.

Also, if someone grabs your hair, you might instinctively reach towards your pain. Again, fight this temptation. Get close, and use your hands to inflict pain on *him* instead.

2. HOLDS. Holds are those restraints aimed at temporarily immobilizing you. They differ from grabs because they require your attacker to use both his hands or arms to restrain you. With your attacker's arms wrapped around you, your arms will either be free (as when he holds you around the waist) or pinned against your sides.

Holds from the rear. If your attacker grabs you from behind and your arms are pinned to your sides, don't try to pry his hands loose, fight against his strength, or struggle to break free. Those responses may all be instinctive, but will accomplish nothing. Instead, go on the offensive and attack his vulnerabilities.

Before you do anything else, however, set your weight. This will help you to stay balanced; it will also make it harder for your attacker to move or pull you in any direction. In fact, if you drop your weight down into a strong and secure stance, your attacker may lose his solid hold on you, briefly freeing your arms and upper body.

And once you've set your weight, cause pain. Nothing will free you faster. Heel-stomp onto his toes or instep, scrape your heel down his shin, or kick your heel straight back into his shin. Or slam your head back hard against his nose. If your hands are pinned tightly to your sides, reach down between his legs and try to grab on. Even if you can't reach his testicles, you can pinch or twist the sensitive skin of his groin and inner thigh. From workshop experience, I can tell you that this hurts like hell. Your attacker will yell or scream, and his hands will move reflexively towards his pain. He will jump back, instinctively recoiling from the cause of the pain.

If you have enough room to move your arm, drive an elbow back hard into his ribs or, better yet, his solar plexus. The solar plexus is a highly vulnerable network of nerves located roughly at the top of the belly—just below the breastbone—where the left and right rib cages meet. (Take a moment to locate it on your own body.)

If your attacker is holding you around your chest or waist, and your arms are free, you have even more options to choose from. For example, you can use your fingers to pinch or twist the skin of his forearms or hands. And don't forget that pinky break: grab hold of his smallest finger and pull it back until you hear it snap.

When an attacker holds you from behind, he's probably bent at the waist and hunched forward "over" you. This puts his face very near to yours. So if you have one arm free, you can elbow-strike backward at his head. Again, take a moment to try this technique yourself. First, make a fist. Second, bend your arm and raise it so your elbow is pointed forward and out, away from your body and parallel to the floor. Now turn (or "torque") at the waist and swing that elbow back and *up* in one forceful, continuous motion. You'll feel for yourself the power that it generates. Just imagine that power connecting with your attacker's jaw, ear, or the side of his head or neck.

The idea is to take advantage of what's available. If you can't use your arms, use your hands. If you can't use your arms or hands, use your legs. If you can't use your arms, hands or legs, use your head or teeth. Forget about what you can't do and concentrate on what you can.

Holds from the front. Holds from the front—or "bear hugs"—offer you different yet equally effective opportunities to inflict pain.

If your arms are pinned to your sides, use your other natural weapons: legs, feet, hands, fingers, head, and (especially) teeth. Bring a knee up between your attacker's legs. Grab for his testicles, or extend your fingers and jab at his groin. Head-butt his nose with the crown of your forehead. Or bite into his shoulder, neck, or cheek as he pulls you close to him. If he tries to kiss you, bite into his lip or tongue.

If your attacker has grabbed you from the front and your arms are *free,* reach up and tear both his ears, or thumb-scrape either one of his eyes. Or go straight to a vital-target attack. Strike or grab his throat, or drive your thumb into his eye.

3. CHOKES. Choking is one of the most frightening things someone can experience during an attack. With someone's hands or arm wrapped around your throat, panic is a common reaction, and for good reason. Choking can threaten your air supply and the oxygen supply to your brain. You may only have a few seconds before you're rendered unconscious, so you must react *immediately.*

Never try to fight against your attacker's strength to break free of a choke. Never try to pull his hands or arm away. Instead, cause pain, and do it fast.

Chokes from the front. If the choke comes from the front—with your attacker facing you—get as close to him as you can so you can inflict pain. If he's choking you at arm's length (with his arms extended stiffly), pinch or twist the skin and hair under his bicep or upper arm. Or place both your hands on the inside crook of his elbow and pull it down and towards you. This will loosen his grip, put him slightly off balance, and bring him close to you. And once he's close, cause serious pain. This man has just tried to choke you, so don't waste time with attention-getters: go straight to a vital-target attack.

Chokes from behind. If an attacker chokes you from behind with his hands, don't try to pull away. Instead, stay as close to him as possible and reach back towards his vulnerable areas. Pinch, twist, grab, or strike his groin area. Stomp down on his instep, scrape your heel against his shin, kick back into his shin, or drive an elbow back into his ribs or solar plexus.

If your attacker is choking you with an arm wrapped around your throat, fight the instinct to pull his arm out and away. Instead, stay close, bring your hands up, and hang on to his arm. Use your body weight to pull it down and towards your chest. As you do this, turn your chin towards the crux of his elbow; this will give you space to breathe. Then cause pain by biting his forearm or using any of the other techniques described above.

The Hidden Advantage: Making "Disadvantages" Work for You

If you're like most women, you've never witnessed an actual fight, only the choreographed "slugfests"—invariably between men—staged for movies and TV. And because men tend to fight in conventional ways, you may have gotten the idea that if you find yourself in certain situations—on the ground, "cornered," or backed against a wall—it means that you're in trouble. In fact, these situations have certain advantages which you can easily exploit.

1. WALL-FIGHTING. Wall-fighting means just that: fighting when pushed or backed against a wall. Most people live in dread of this situation; in their minds, it's synonymous with being trapped and helpless. After all, the expression "backed against a wall" is used to describe situations where one literally or figuratively has no escape route.

In fact, fighting actually becomes easier when you're backed up against a wall, or, for that matter, a door, post, fence, car, or high railing. Why should this be so? Simple—support. Anytime you have a solid structure behind you, it gives you added support. You can't be pushed backwards off your feet, and the chances of you slipping, tripping, or being shoved or pushed to the ground are dramatically reduced. And that support from a solid structure can be crucial if you happen to be elderly, pregnant, injured, or have some physical weakness (bad back, weak knees, etc.).

Wall-fighting has such advantages that I encourage you to deliberately back yourself up against a solid structure if an attacker is approaching and a fight seems inevitable. If this seems like a contradiction of my earlier advice to move towards your attacker, it really isn't. Remember, I also encouraged you to fight smart, and purposely putting a solid structure behind you can be the smarter way to go. Back up slowly, and you let your attacker think he has you right where he wants you. By retreating, you've made him think that you're afraid. In fact, you're the one who's really in control. You know that once you find that wall, its extra support will help you fight back more effectively.

Supportive structures also serve as great weapons. For example, after you've hooked the back of your attacker's neck and pushed your thumb into his eye, use your non-action hand to bang his head against the wall behind you. Bang it repeatedly and you can render your attacker unconscious.

Finally, if your back is against a wall, it ensures that no one can approach you from behind. Attacks by multiple attackers are rare, but there's always the chance that your attacker has a companion or companions with him. With your back against a wall, you can see everything and everyone around you.

2. CORNER-FIGHTING. This means fighting while backed into the corner of a room, stairwell, garage, or basically any location where two walls meet. And once again, what is commonly perceived as a disadvantage ("I've got you cornered") is actually a plus. All the advantages of wall-fighting apply to corner-fighting as well, with one additional benefit: corner-fighting gives you a second wall to use as a weapon in a fight.

3. GROUND-FIGHTING. There's no getting around it: many attacks end up on the ground, especially attempted rapes. You might slip or trip in a physical scuffle, or your attacker might drag or shove you off your feet.

This doesn't mean you're finished, however; it just means it's time to switch tactics. So don't panic. Believe it or not, the ground is one of the *safest* places to be when engaged in a fight. With the support of the ground beneath you, you can't be injured by falling, tripping, or being shoved off your feet.

The key to successful self-defense when you're on the ground is to *fight from that position*. The worst mistake you can make—and one most people make instinctively—is to try to get up. Don't do this! Stay on the ground. If you're attacked while in bed, stay on the bed. Use gravity to your advantage, not his. So never try to get up, push up, or lift your arms. Never struggle against an attacker's weight on top of you. Remember, you want to conserve your energy. Struggling to get up will only waste that energy in a futile attempt to escape a stronger, *uninjured* attacker.

If you're attacked on the ground, your attacker will probably straddle your waist with his knees while he pins you down at the wrists or arms. In this position, he's as balanced as a four-legged table. And with his weight on top of you, it's only natural to feel trapped. Whenever I conduct a workshop and have a woman pinned down in this fashion, I see the fear and helplessness in her eyes. Indeed, most of the women I've trained describe this scenario as the one they fear most.

There's still no reason to panic, however. There isn't much your attacker can do while his hands are holding you down. So be patient; you can stay there all day if you want to. And remember: the moment he releases his hold on one or both of your arms, he will become as imbalanced and unstable as a three-legged table. And however frightening it may feel, the very fact that your attacker is "all over you" is to your advantage: it means vital targets are more accessible than they might be if you were fighting on your feet.

To attack those vital targets, however, you must get at least one of your hands free. There are two ways you can accomplish this. You can either take the initiative and make him release your arm, or you can wait for him to let go.

Taking the Initiative

If you want to make the first move, the following techniques are designed to make your attacker release one or both of your arms.

- Yell at the top of your lungs. Your attacker may put a hand over your mouth to quiet you, thereby freeing one of your arms.
- Turn your head and sink your teeth into his hand, wrist, or forearm. He'll pull away from your bite, giving you one free hand. His healthy arm may even move towards his injury, giving you *two* free hands.
- If your attacker tries to kiss you on the mouth, bite into his lip, tongue, or cheek. As he recoils from the pain, one of his hands will instinctively move towards his injury.
- Shoot your arms up above your head, keeping your arms on the ground *at all times*. This will drag your attacker's hands and knuckles along the ground. If you're lying on

concrete or gravel, this can inflict enough pain to get a quick release. (It can even work on carpeting.) This technique also disrupts your attacker's balance because his weight is on your arms.

- Straighten one of your arms up above your head while you simultaneously straighten your other arm down towards your hip. (Keep both arms on the ground as you drag them; never try to lift them.) Do this in a quick movement; surprise and speed are essential. You will immediately unsettle your attacker's balance. He'll try to "catch" himself, and you'll be able to free one or both of your arms.

Waiting for Your Moment

If your intuition is telling you to wait and let your attacker make the first move, that's fine, too; he has to make a move eventually. So stay calm, and be patient. Tell him that you won't fight back, that you'll do "whatever he wants." Put him at ease. Then, when he inevitably moves a hand down to lift up your skirt, take off your pants, or take off his pants, you'll have the one free hand you need to fight. As your attacker releases one or both of your arms to proceed with his assault, his body will also lift up, again unsettling his balance. He is now extremely vulnerable to counter-attack.

Once you reach the point where you have one or both of your arms free, you're ready to cause pain. And of all the different ground-fighting techniques you can choose from, I believe that going for the eye is by far the most effective. An attack to the groin or throat, however devastating, may cause your attacker to collapse on top of you, impeding your escape. When you attack his eye, however, you control his head, and where the head goes, the body goes. You'll be able to turn his head and direct his body off of you. So whenever possible, go after the eye when fighting from the ground.

The moment you get one hand free, therefore, immediately hook the neck of your attacker. This instruction may surprise you; you might be wondering why I don't advise causing pain with that hand. Here's why: if you hurt your attacker with your free hand, he will move away from that hand, then re-trap it using his weight and leverage.

If you use your free hand to hook the back of his neck, however, you'll put your attacker off balance and control his entire body. As you pull him down towards you, he'll instinctively release his grip on your other arm in an attempt to catch himself. Even if his grip is only weakened, you should be able to get your other hand free and drive your thumb into his eye.

You attack the eye in exactly the same way as you would if you were standing up. First, hook the back of his neck and pull it down into your shoulder. (If you hook with your left hand, bring his head to your left shoulder; if you hook it with your right hand, bring his head to your right shoulder.) Then drive the thumb of your other hand forcefully into his eye. At the same time, grip the side of his temple as though you're trying to make a fist, keep your elbows in, and *don't let up the pressure*. Expect to hear screams or cries of pain, and expect to feel him struggle. These reactions mean your attack is working!

If you can't reach your attacker's neck to hook it because his upper body is erect, drive a hammer fist down onto his bladder or groin. The pain will cause him to reflexively double at the waist and drop his head towards you.

Once you hook the back of your attacker's neck and attack his eye, it will become very easy to get him off you. Without loosening your grip, and with your elbows tucked in tight, use your action (attacking) hand to turn his head; his body will twist in the same direction. Then, as you turn his head, plant a foot on the ground and push off as you rotate your hips. If your right hand is attacking his eye, push off with your right foot; if your left hand is attacking, push off with your left foot.

As he topples over to one side, maintain your hold and roll with him. Now you're lying on your side with your thumb still in his eye and your other hand still behind his neck. Keep your elbows in and bounce his head off the ground. If you're on a hard surface—sidewalk, tarmac, or uncarpeted floor—so much the better: just like a wall, the ground can serve as an excellent secondary weapon.

Once the fight has gone out of your attacker, it's time to get rid of him. (And believe me, you'll know when he's finished.)

Shove him away with both your open palms, then sit up and pivot on your buttocks so your feet are pointed in his direction. Use your hands to slide away from him along the floor. That way, if he makes a last-ditch lunge towards you, you can heel-kick out or axe-kick down to his groin, chest, face, or ribs. Don't try to get up until you've immobilized him, gotten clear of his reach, and know you can get to safety.

One final thought on ground-fighting. Much to my dismay, there are some popular self-defense programs that teach women to *deliberately* drop to the ground when confronted by an attacker. Their logic goes that since a woman's legs are the most powerful parts of her body, she should endeavor to fight from a seated position and kick her attacker's legs, groin, or head. In my opinion, encouraging anyone to deliberately drop to the ground in an assault situation is just plain bad advice, and for several reasons. One, it immediately reduces your options; you can't do anything else *but* kick. Two, it demands a certain level of physical agility to pivot on your rear end and keep your legs pointed towards a moving attacker. Three, if you're on the ground, you can't get close to your attacker and cause pain: you have to wait for him to get close to you. And while you're waiting, there's nothing to stop him from hurling a heavy object (rock, brick, chair, you name it) in your direction.

If you're pushed, shoved or forced to the ground, by all means fight from the ground. Otherwise, stay on your feet: it's always preferable to fight from a rooted and balanced position. With your feet planted firmly on the ground, you can use *all* your natural weapons to bring an attacker to his knees. And running to safety is a heck of a lot easier when you're standing than when you're lying on your back!

4. SEATED-FIGHTING. One of the most inspiring people I've met in my martial arts study is a fellow student named Bill. A third degree black belt, Bill is confined to a wheelchair. Although he has no legs, Bill is a tremendous fighter with incredible heart and stamina. And he's living proof that you can fight from a seated position.

A woman can be attacked while seated at a desk, on a park

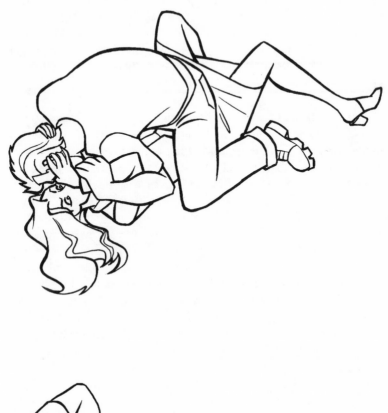

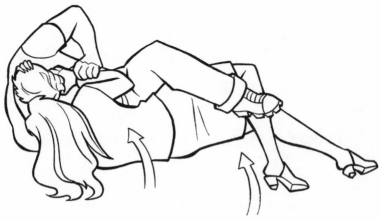

Getting out from under an attacker [steps 1 *(top)* and 2]

bench, on a bus or subway train, or behind the wheel of her car. If you're attacked while seated, your instinctive reaction will probably be to try to stand up. But as with ground-fighting, this is usually a futile exercise, wasting precious energy. Your strength will be no match for the combined forces of gravity and your attacker's weight. So forget about getting up. Do what Bill does: fight from a seated position, zeroing in on accessible targets.

When an attacker stands over you, his bladder and groin are particularly accessible; they're literally right in front of you. If you drop a solid hammer fist down on either target, you can drop him to his knees. At the very least, he will double over, bringing vulnerable targets like his ears, throat, and eyes within your reach.

In many situations, you can use what you're sitting on as a secondary weapon. As you hook the back of your attacker's neck and attack his eye, for example, slam his head straight down onto the arm of your chair or bench. If you're in your car, use the steering wheel or dashboard. When Bill works out at the studio, he uses the arm rests and metal frame of his wheelchair as secondary weapons. Or he propels his chair into his opponent's shin, or over his opponent's toes.

I've never had to fight from a wheelchair, but I've learned two valuable lessons from Bill. First, that heart and desire mean absolutely everything when it comes to surmounting seemingly impossible obstacles. Second, that fighting from a seated position is not only possible, but has particular advantages. Thanks, Bill.

"Sticks and Stones"

Physical attacks are nearly always accompanied by some form of verbal assault. Yelling, threats, and offensive language are part of any aggressor's arsenal, and he uses them as he would a knife, a gun, or any other weapon: to intimidate and control his victim. Meanwhile, the need to humiliate and degrade isn't confined to rapists and attackers; it's also the driving force behind most sexual harassment, street harassment, and hate crimes.

We all know the schoolyard rhyme, "Sticks and stones may break my bones, but words will never hurt me." But if they cannot "break your bones," words can still do damage. They can shock and intimidate you. They can break your spirit and tear down your resistance. They can compromise your very ability to fight. *So you need to be prepared for them.*

"Bitch," "whore," and "slut" (or worse) aren't words in my vocabulary; just *writing* them makes me uncomfortable. But they're precisely the kind of words harassers and attackers use against their victims. Fortunately, the more familiar you become with this kind of language, the less power and shock value it will have. So read those words again. Say them aloud. And remember: they don't apply to you in any way, shape, or form.

Because I want my students to be prepared for anything and everything, I try to make our role-playing exercises as realistic as possible. So when I play the part of an attacker or harasser, I always use degrading, offensive language. I yell insults, obscenities, vulgarities: the harsher, more abusive, and louder the better. And time and again, I see the effect that mere words can have on the human psyche. Some women are so startled and shocked by my language, they actually forget to fight or otherwise assert themselves. Others are embarrassed and humiliated; I've seen many fight back tears. Still others become downright angry. Yet as painful as this exercise may be for some students, it has two important benefits: they learn to expect abusive language, and then become enured to it. When it comes to offensive language, familiarity literally breeds contempt.

To a significant degree, self-esteem plays a role in how we react to verbal coercion. Invariably, the poorer a student's self-esteem, the more likely she is to become humiliated, embarrassed, upset, and hurt by abusive language. By contrast, students with stronger self-esteem are more likely to respond with a healthy, "Who do you think you're talking to?!" attitude. Ideally, of course, neither a person's words nor the volume of his voice should have any effect on you. But if you're going to react emotionally, I'd rather see you respond with indignation than with embarrassment, shock, or hurt. Properly channeled, anger can empower you. After all, "I'm mad as hell . . ." goes hand in hand with ". . . and I'm not going to take it anymore!"

"The Seducer"

Throughout *The Odyssey,* the epic tale of Ulysses' voyage home from Troy, Ulysses encountered many hazards. These included the Sirens, whose song was so sweet and so bewitching it lured sailors to their doom upon the rocks.

Equally bewitching is the "song" of the aggressor who uses words to reassure, persuade, and seduce his victim. This approach is the norm for most harassers, but it's also used by many rapists. The seductive rapist takes an altogether different approach from one who hurls threats and abusive language, but his intentions are just the same *and he is every bit as dangerous.* The seductive rapist can be very convincing. His victim may actually start to believe that everything really *will* "be all right" if she just does as she's told, cooperates, plays along. Yet every reassurance comes with the implicit or explicit threat of violence:

- "I'm not going to hurt you *(. . . but I can if I want to)."*
- "I don't want to hurt you *(. . . but I will if you resist)."*
- "Think about your kids *(. . . or you'll never see them again)."*
- "Don't make me mad *(. . . or you will be badly hurt or killed)."*

Metaphorically speaking, the abusive rapist uses the whip, while the seductive rapist uses the carrot. He dangles the promise of his victim's survival right before her very eyes. Often, he uses the actual language of seduction, as though he is not really a rapist but an admirer, lover, or friend:

- "You're going to enjoy this."
- "You're so beautiful, I can't help myself."
- "Relax. Don't be so cold/frigid/mean."

And so on. Sometimes this romantic approach is an act, but sometimes it isn't; in many cases, the rapist may not think of himself as a rapist. (This is especially true in an acquaintance or date rape where he already knows the woman.) Whatever he may say, however, and however sweetly he may say it, you should respond as forcefully against the seducer as you would against any attacker.

Now that you know what to expect, let's take another look at the kind of things the seducer may say, but this time, imagine how you might *mentally* respond to them:

Him	*You*
"I don't want to hurt you."	Yes, you do: you want to rape me.
"I'm not going to hurt you."	You've got that right: I'm going to hurt *you*.
"Think about your kids."	I am thinking about them. That's why *you're* in trouble.
"Don't make me mad."	Your anger doesn't frighten me.

In *The Odyssey,* Ulysses stuffed his men's ears with wax so they wouldn't hear the Sirens' voices. And when it comes to the seductive rapist, understanding his modus operandi will enable you to avoid the trap he tries to set.

9
WORST-CASE SCENARIOS

Although many rapes and assaults are carried out by a lone, unarmed attacker, that isn't always the case. You may have to face an assailant armed with a knife or gun, or multiple attackers. Or you may find yourself in a situation which seems to confirm your deepest fears, in which resistance suddenly seems futile. Fortunately, whatever the situation, you nearly always have options. And as you will see, some of them are very effective.

When it comes to violent assault, I want you to be prepared for anything and everything. There is a difference, however, between being prepared and being paranoid, between living smart and living in fear. So even as we examine some of the "worst-case scenarios" of violent assault, bear one thing in mind: they *do* represent exceptions to the rule. From a purely statistical standpoint, the chances are good that you will never encounter them.

Multiple Attackers

National crime statistics confirm that the vast majority of rapes are committed by a lone individual; only a very small minority of women are attacked by two or more assailants. As rare as the multiple attacker scenario is, however, it can and does occur, and it's better to be safe than sorry. Fortunately, fighting off two or more people is easier than you may think.

In most action and martial arts movies, there comes a point when the hero is confronted by multiple attackers. And as surely as the sun will rise in the east, you can bet that he'll fight them all simultaneously. He'll punch one bad guy, kick another, then go back to the first guy to finish him off. And so on. It's all very impressive, very exciting . . . and totally unrealistic.

Just how unrealistic was something I learned from experience. The simultaneous, multiple-attacker attack is one of the things that San Soo students train for: just when they become comfortable fighting one-on-one, the instructor will ask them to train in "threes." Each student takes turns fighting off two "attackers." And the first time I tried this, I made the classic mistake: I tried to fight them both simultaneously. As a result, I didn't fight either one of them effectively.

There are two fundamental principles of fighting multiple attackers. First, you must go after them one at a time; you can't fight two people at once. Second, you must go on the offensive.

Let's say you're walking to your car one night when you're suddenly confronted by two men. You believe that you are about to be attacked, and physical resistance seems your only recourse. What do you do?

Although we've already discussed the importance of fighting offensively, that principle becomes *doubly* important when fighting two or more people. Going on the offensive will put you in control of the situation. It will surprise your attackers—it's the last thing they expect—and put them at a disadvantage. Attackers operating with a partner or in a group are usually bolder and more aggressive than a lone assailant, and unlikely to be deterred by such stall tactics as verbal resistance or negotiation. And at all costs, you want to prevent a situation in which two or more people are restraining you.

Therefore, if an attack by multiple assailants seems inevitable, and your best option is physical resistance, *don't wait* for them to make the first move. Go after the man closest to you, and do it fast. Attacker #1 has got to experience extreme pain right away. If you choose to use an attention-getter, you've got to make it count. I prefer to go after vital targets only, especially the eye. Of all the techniques you can choose from, the eye attack seems to work best when dealing with multiple attackers. First, it enables you to inflict great pain and damage quickly. Before he knows what's happening, Attacker #1 is in big trouble: he's in pain but cannot break free from your grasp. Second, this technique allows you to control Attacker #1 *and use him as a barrier between you and his accomplice.* This is an extremely important concept. You always want to keep someone between you and the other attacker(s). And with his head pulled down and into your chest, Attacker #1 is basically trapped. With your hooking hand wrapped behind his neck and your thumb in his eye, you'll be able to move him around into any position you like.

So as soon as you grab Attacker #1, use him as a shield. Continue doing so until you can get rid of him and move on to Attacker #2. And that's precisely what you need to do: *go after the next guy.* Don't wait for him to make a move towards you. You've put his partner out of commission, and now you're going to end this once and for all.

All you're doing is what I've trained you to do: fight one-on-one. The only difference is that you're now doing it in sequence, going after one attacker, then another, and (if necessary) yet another. Suddenly, two against one or three against one becomes *one* against one. You may be facing multiple attackers, but it's no longer a multiple attack.

And don't underestimate the pain and damage you will inflict on Attacker #1. Eye attacks can be devastating, and the more devastating your initial attack, the better. Believe me, Attacker #2 is less likely to intercede or press his attack if he hears his friend screaming and sees you inflicting serious pain and injury.

In any situation involving multiple attackers, you should also try to back into a corner, or against a wall or other solid structure. In addition to giving you support, this reduces the chance that you'll be attacked simultaneously from the front and rear.

Remember: fighting off two or more attackers can be accomplished if you forget about trying to run away or struggle free and think "attack" at all times. Nothing works quite as well as turning the tables on others who want to hurt you.

Attackers with Weapons

If the only information you get on rape and assaults is from the media, it's easy to get the impression that nearly all rapes and assaults are carried out with weapons. In fact, actual crime statistics tell quite another story. For example, because you're far more likely to be raped by someone you know than by a stranger—and most "acquaintance rapists" are unarmed—the majority of rapes are committed with no weapon at all.

Of course, that kind of statistic is cold comfort to anyone who has faced a knife-wielding rapist, or been robbed at gunpoint. And I have yet to hold a seminar without having at least one person ask me what to do if an attacker has a knife or gun. The possibility frightens most people, and understandably so: an armed attacker *is* more dangerous than an unarmed one, and criminals are more likely to be armed today than ever before. So while I want to emphasize that the odds are in your favor that you'll never face an armed assailant, you should still know what action to take—and *not* take—just in case you do. As the saying goes, forewarned *is* forearmed.

The Power of Persuasion

Any assailant who brandishes a weapon does so for one very simple reason: it makes his job easier. If he can intimidate his victim, she'll be more compliant and less likely to resist. If causing pain is "the great equalizer" for a woman confronted by a larger, stronger male aggressor, a gun or knife tips the odds heavily in that aggressor's favor even if he never uses it. The intimidation factor of knives and guns is enormous. Most people are deathly afraid of them, and it's that fear which the armed attacker counts on. He actually uses your fear of his weapon—rather than the weapon itself—in order to control you.

Nonresistance

If an armed assailant demands your purse, your jewelry, even your car, don't think twice about handing it over. Place your personal safety over *any* material possession. At the same time, do everything you can to de-escalate the situation. The more nervous or edgy an assailant is, the more dangerous he is, so try to keep him calm. Keep your voice low and even. Whatever you do, don't scream. Tell him you'll give him "whatever he wants"; convince him of your compliance. And don't make any sudden movements: if you have to reach into your pocket or purse, for example, do it slowly, and warn him ahead of time. Keep your hands where he can see them. Remember that most armed muggers have no intention of killing their victim. If they did, they wouldn't waste time with threats and verbal coercion.

I would also urge nonresistance at least initially in some rape and assault situations involving a weapon. The presence of a gun or knife always demands an extra degree of caution, and sometimes (though not always), the best thing to do is be patient. Wait for an opening or opportunity—when your attacker drops his guard, or lays his weapon aside—before you make your move.

In deciding whether or not to resist an armed attacker, always let your intuition be your guide. If your inner voice is telling you not to resist, then don't. But if your intuition is warning you, "I'm going to be hurt whether I comply or not," then you may want to make the choice to fight.

The Armed Rapist

Most law enforcement personnel will tell you to always comply with the demands of an armed assailant: no if's, and's, or but's. I agree with this advice if your assailant "only" intends to rob you. I do believe, however, that active resistance is appropriate—and even essential—in certain situations. Most of these involve the armed rapist.

I've had some women tell me, "I'd rather die than allow myself to be raped," while others say that they would endure the trauma of rape in order to escape with their life. Neither one of these responses is right or wrong, of course. The choice to fight an armed rapist is yours and yours alone.

At the same time you should know that, statistically speaking, some situations involving an armed rapist are more dangerous than others. If he attempts to force you to a secondary location—especially into a car—your life could easily be in danger. The same is true if he tries to handcuff you or tie you up, or if the rape attempt occurs not in a public place but in your home; generally, the more isolated the location, the greater the risk to your life.

Many experts on rape distinguish between different "types" of rapists: the insecure, the sadistic, the self-centered, and so on. (FBI profiler John Douglas differentiates between the "power assurance rapist" and the "anger excitation" rapist.) Many times, a woman is urged to adopt a self-defense strategy appropriate to the rapist's personality type. For example, if the rapist is the insecure type, she is told that things like negotiation and verbal self-defense might very well deter him; if he is the sadistic type, however, she is warned that those same tactics are likely to enrage him and spur him to greater violence.

Unfortunately, no matter what personality type he may appear to conform to, it's my firm belief that *any rapist has the potential to be sadistic*. In the blink of an eye, the rapist who initially seems nervous and insecure may turn vicious. Therefore, your self-defense strategy must remain flexible, ready to change from moment to moment. My advice is that you operate on the assumption that your rapist is the sadistic type, and work back from there. If he turns out to be the insecure type, fine. But I'd rather see you expect the worst even as you hope for the best.

If you feel nonresistance may save your life, then follow that path. But if you feel that your attacker intends to *use* his weapon, then resist with all the confidence and determination you can muster. Though their stories rarely make the evening news, many women do escape armed rapists: sometimes by fighting back, yet sometimes by using nothing but their wits. Remember, the armed rapist rarely expects you to resist, and that gives you an advantage.

Surprisingly, my workshop experience has taught me that it's actually very difficult to rape a woman while holding onto a weapon. Consider for a moment all that a rapist must accomplish with just one hand: grab hold of his victim, get her on the ground, pin her down, drop his pants and underwear, remove her pants or push up her skirt, and remove her underwear. It's no easy task.

Sometimes, of course, the armed rapist will force his victim to do much of this work herself, threatening her with bodily harm or death if she doesn't comply. Whether he performs these tasks himself, however, or forces his victim to perform them, there comes a point in many rapes when the armed rapist lays his weapon aside. This is especially true if the woman has not screamed, struggled, or otherwise tried to resist. I know one woman who was attacked by a knife-wielding rapist in her college dorm room. Megan initially chose not to fight back. As her attacker pushed her on the bed and began groping her with his free hand, however, she promised to comply with his every demand if he would "just put down the knife." Her tactic worked; her attacker actually laid the knife on the nightstand. And the moment he did, Megan kneed him right between his legs, inflicting enough pain that she was able to break free and escape.

An unarmed rapist is especially vulnerable to counterattack. Because he's all over his "victim," at least one of his vital targets—eyes, throat, or testicles—is well within her reach.

Active Resistance

What if your attacker never lays his weapon aside, yet you choose to fight back? Your options are more limited with armed attackers than with unarmed ones, but they do exist. Some strategies are appropriate only to guns, others only to knives. However, there are two principles to keep in mind for virtually *any* type of weapon:

#1: Don't focus on the weapon itself, or try to wrestle it from your attacker. A gun or knife is harmless without the hand to fire or wield it, so focus on the hand, the arm, the *person*.

#2: If your attacker drops his weapon or lays it aside, *don't go after it.* Instead, go after your attacker. Now that he's unarmed, you meet on a level playing field.

Guns

Many years ago, an instructor pointed a gun at me during a private training session. Though it looked exactly like the real thing it was just a pellet gun, and of course it wasn't loaded. But if it posed no actual threat to my life, it still terrified me. When you're looking down the barrel of a gun—real or not, loaded or unloaded—it looks like a cannon. You can't take your eyes off it. The feeling is surreal. When my instructor pointed it at my stomach, I actually felt a pain in my gut and I instinctively took a step back. If a fake gun could illicit this reaction, imagine what it's like to confront the real thing.

There's not much room for forgiveness when a gun is pointed right at you. A gunshot wound can easily be fatal; therefore, the decision to fight an attacker who has a gun must never be made lightly. It really must be reserved for situations where your life is on the line. It just baffles me when I read about a motorist killed after resisting the demands of an armed carjacker; to risk one's life for a BMW is utterly senseless.

If you do choose to fight someone who has a gun, you can only do so if you're close to him. If the gun is pointed at you from any distance, fighting is simply not an option; you're just too far away. Get close to your attacker, however, and you can control his weapon hand and cause pain simultaneously. Remember: you can't be shot by a gun unless it's pointed *right at you*. You only need to deflect the barrel a few inches, therefore, to put you out of the line of fire.

Before you do this, however, you must first establish physical contact with the weapon hand. This is accomplished by gently, I repeat, *gently* touching the inside of his wrist; a gentle touch to the wrist is perceived as nonthreatening, if it is noticed at all. By contrast, a sudden, jittery grab of his wrist might easily startle him into firing his weapon. Then, when you're ready to make your move, grab his wrist tightly and deflect the gun barrel out and away from you; move his weapon hand in one direction while you simultaneously move your body in the opposite direction. And the instant you're clear of the barrel of the gun, CAUSE PAIN. Grab his windpipe, scrape his eye, knee him in the testicles, anything to inflict serious pain and damage. Keep in mind that your goal is not to get possession of the gun, but to make him lose possession. As soon as the gun is out of his hand, it cannot hurt you. That's the moment when *all* of your attention should shift towards the man.

Believe it or not, running from an attacker who has a gun is also an option in certain situations. It's not that easy to hit a moving target, especially if it is dark outside and especially if you duck and weave. Police officers are trained in the use of firearms, yet they miss all the time.

In making the decision to run, distance should be the determining factor. It certainly was for Leslie. While in a supermarket parking lot, placing groceries in the trunk of her car, she saw a man heading towards her with a gun in his hand. He was about 10 yards away, so she decided to run for it. She felt the chances of him shooting her in the back were pretty remote, and for several reasons: it was dark out, there were other people around, and her intuition told her that he was more intent on robbery than homicide. Her judgment turned out to be accurate; no shots were fired as she fled back inside the market.

Knives

Most people will say that they'd rather be shot with a gun than stabbed with a knife. Never mind that guns are the weapon of choice in many homicides; the fear of being stabbed by a sharp object is so universal it's almost primal.

While a gun is only dangerous when it's pointed directly at you, the same cannot be said for knives. You can be cut or stabbed by a knife inadvertently: in a struggle, or when your attacker recoils from pain. And some inadvertent knife wounds—however quick, however superficial—can literally be fatal. To understand why this is so, it helps to understand the vulnerabilities of the human body.

The most vulnerable parts of your body are those responsible for major blood flow. Fortunately, some of these areas (such as your heart and aorta) are fairly well-protected from inadvertent (read: superficial) knife wounds. Meanwhile, other areas are more accessible, but easy to repair; bleeding from the radial artery, for example (as when someone slashes a wrist), is fairly easy to staunch. It's in the area of the neck where your jugular veins, carotid arteries, and windpipe are close to the surface that inadvertent knife wounds pose the greatest threat to your life. Always move with extreme caution if a knife is held against or near to your throat. Make any sudden movements, and you might trigger a wound that could actually be fatal.

Because you can be cut by a knife inadvertently, it's essential that you know where it is *at all times*. And as with a gun, you should determine where the knife is by making gentle contact with the weapon hand; any sudden movement might cause you to be cut or stabbed, even as your attacker tries to pull away from you. And once you have contact—once you "know" where his knife is—CAUSE PAIN. As long as you're controlling his weapon hand, you won't be inadvertently cut as he recoils in pain. Remember, *always fight the man, not the weapon,* so never try to wrestle the knife away without first causing pain.

If your attacker is facing you, deflect his knife hand out and away in one direction as you move your body in another while you simultaneously cause pain. However, if your attacker is behind you with his knife held near the front of your throat, tighten your grip on his weapon hand and hang on it. You want to use your body weight to pull it down and *close* against your chest, making that weapon hand a "part" of you. With attacks from the rear, you want to deprive your attacker of any leverage, so fight the natural instinct to push or pull his knife hand away from your body. Holding his weapon hand close against your body immobilizes it. Try as he might, he won't be able to cut you.

Next, cause pain with an attention-getter: drive your heel down onto his instep or toes, scrape your heel down his shin, drive your elbow back into his ribs, reach back and grab his testicles, or hammer-strike his testicles with your fist. Your goal is to make him focus on his pain (and perhaps loosen his grip on his weapon) long enough for you to turn and face him. Alternatively, you can also *wait* for him to turn you round. The point is this: once you're facing him, you can attack one of his vital targets. You can drive a knee up between his legs, scrape your thumb across his eye, or wrap your hand behind his neck, pull him towards you, and sink your teeth into his windpipe. **Note:** You can do any one of these things with just one free hand. This is important, because whether your attacker is behind you or in front of you, you should not let go of his weapon hand as you cause pain. I want you to fight offensively and with total commitment, but you must maintain control over the weapon hand at all times.

Fighting anyone who has a knife always involves some risk. Sanford Strong recounts the chilling yet inspiring story of a woman attacked as she walked down a secluded path. Her attacker wore a nylon stocking over his face. When he pulled out a knife, she decided that he was more than "just" a rapist, that he meant to cut and possibly kill her. *So she grabbed the blade of the knife.* Although her hand was badly injured, her gutsy move enabled her to fight her way to safety.

I share her story to make one final point: that in any struggle with an attacker armed with a knife, total commitment is essential. You must be willing to risk pain and minor injury in order to avoid major injury and death. You have to move beyond your fear of the pain and say to yourself, "Even though I might get cut, I've got to fight."

"But What If . . . ?": Confronting Our Worst Fears

Anytime I address an audience on the subject of self-defense, I inevitably meet some level of resistance to my ideas. Usually, this takes the form of a "but what if . . ." question, as in, "I understand what you're saying, *but what if* my attacker has a gun?" or "I could fight off one guy, *but what if* there are two of them?" Over time, I've come to expect this kind of response. I believe that in the back of most people's minds, there's at least one situation where resistance would be futile and escape impossible.

I'm the first person to admit that self-defense training has its limitations. While it does increase your odds of survival, you can't expect it to protect you all the time, in every situation. Yet I'm also convinced that many of the situations people perceive to be hopeless aren't necessarily so. We've already discussed two of these in depth: those involving multiple attackers and attackers with weapons. I've also explained how some situations that appear to put you at a disadvantage (pinned to the ground, for example, or backed against a wall) actually give you definite advantages. Now it's time to "emphasize the positive" in some other situations you may fear the most.

- **Being ambushed or taken by surprise.** Throughout this book, I've offered many suggestions about what to do if an aggressor is approaching you and an attack seems inevitable: set your weight, for example, or get a solid structure behind you. But what if you don't have the chance to do anything at all? What if your attacker comes out of nowhere so suddenly and explosively that you haven't time to react (much less act) before you're tackled to the ground? This is a very real possibility. In his book, *Journey Into Darkness,* John Douglas describes one serial rapist who perfected a "blitz" style of attack, ambushing his victims from behind as they exited city buses. Douglas also describes situations where women and teenage girls have been kidnapped off the street—in broad daylight, no less, and sometimes in crowded areas—by one or more attackers. A car pulls up alongside with two men inside; one acts as a lookout while the other jumps out, grabs the woman, and drags her into the car. Boom: it's over in a matter of seconds.

I believe that the surprise attack that a woman fears the most is the one that occurs inside her home, especially late at night and while she is asleep. A woman awakens to find an attacker pinning her to the bed, possibly with a knife held to her throat. Her initial disorientation gives way to panic. She doesn't have time to yell for help, call 911, or get to a weapon even if she has one in the house. Her attacker uses the very privacy of her own home to isolate her and place her under his control.

And it's true: anyone who breaks into your home while you are there poses a serious threat. Burglars are only interested in your possessions, so they choose to enter your home when you're not there. Home intruders, on the other hand, are often looking to hurt you, rape you, or worse. Sanford Strong cites statistics showing that a person is six times more likely to be killed during an armed home intrusion than during a street mugging or robbery; one particular study concluded that 35 percent of home intrusions result in serious injuries or murders. Yet it's also true that no matter where a surprise attack occurs, whether in the home or on the street, it needn't end with the victim's injury or death. Unless her attacker kills her right then and there, a woman always has options, some of them highly effective.

The one thing that may stop her from using those options will be her own fear. That's precisely why mental preparation is so important when it comes to surprise attacks. Instead of hoping for the best, accept the reality that surprise attacks can and do occur, then "rehearse" them in your mind. Be prepared for the fact that you may be tackled to the ground and suffer initial pain and injury.

At the same time, do everything you can in terms of prevention: follow the tips on home security contained in the chapter, "The Safety Factor: Your Personal Daily Checklist," then reread the earlier chapters "An Ounce of Prevention" and "Safety as a Way of Life." Finally, always listen to your intuition. A large percentage of "surprise" attacks are really not that at all: many victims recall feeling nervous or uneasy well before they were attacked.

One final thought. In many surprise attacks, the victim may not actually see her attacker. She may be ambushed from behind, or attacked in the dark; either way, the effect is disorienting and frightening. This need not be the case, however. Fighting is far more dependent on *feel* than on sight. If you can feel your attacker, you can hurt him. It's just that simple. To get this point across, I like to use a "Blindfold Exercise" in my training programs. Once my students have learned how to fight off an attacker, I blindfold them and give them the opportunity to defend themselves without the benefit of eyesight. Although initially apprehensive, my students soon learn that you don't need to see your attacker in order to fight effectively. So even if you're attacked in a pitch-black room or darkened parking garage, or you lose your eyeglasses moments into an attack, forget about your inability to see and rely upon your sense of touch. It's all you really need.

• **Being harassed, threatened, or attacked while you're with your children.** If a woman is out in public with her children, just being approached by a street crazy or harasser can cause her great anxiety. If she were alone, she might not hesitate to respond assertively with boundary-setting or verbal self-defense techniques. But with a child at her side or in her arms, she may be too afraid to do just that. And that fear becomes even greater if she is physically accosted or attacked.

Aggressors know that a child can be a woman's "Achilles' heel," discouraging her from attempting any resistance whatsoever. It's not uncommon for them to use the parental bond to control a woman, so you should never assume that a child's presence will necessarily discourage harassment or attack. And anytime you're with a person who depends on you for their safety—an infant, small child, or even an older parent—it's true that you have to exercise an extra degree of caution.

However, there's a real difference between acting cautiously, and taking no action at all. And whether you're alone or with your children, *the basic principles of self-defense remain the same.* I've explained, for example, that because most rapists test a woman's boundaries for signs of weakness, stepping forward and using verbal self-defense is not a form of risk-taking but is actually the *safer* way to go. When it comes to physical attacks, I've explained why getting close, going on the offensive, and causing pain are your best means of protection. Just remember: these principles hold true even when there's a small child by your side.

As soon as they're old enough to learn it, we teach our children about fire safety. We teach them how to dial 911. We emphasize how important it is that they exit a burning building quickly and calmly; we may even teach them how to crawl on hands and knees to avoid inhaling smoke. I bring this up to illustrate that even a small child can be taught what to do in a crisis. And when it comes to harassment and especially assault, children can and should know how to help you and help themselves. Role-playing is a great way to get this across; most children love to pretend. For example, you might say, "If I told you to run for help, what would you do?" Depending on the situation, the correct answer might be to run to the next-door neighbor, or to a phone to dial 911. I think some kind of rehearsal is important; without it, your children may be unable to respond in a crisis. They may be too confused or frightened to follow your commands. Yet whether a child goes for help or not, running, period, is usually their best defense.

In recent years, carjacking has become yet another threat we have to worry about, and there have been several well-publicized cases where armed carjackers have stolen or tried to steal a woman's car with her children still strapped inside. If a carjacker has a gun (and most do), I don't believe that physical resistance is an option. You might be able to deflect the gun barrel away from you, only to have it pointed at your child. Therefore, your best option is to use a combination of nonresistance, de-escalation, and clear communication. Tell him he can have the car, no questions asked (nonresistance). Don't shriek, scream, or make any sudden movements; instead, keep your voice calm and low and your body language nonthreatening (de-escalation). At the same time, say, "I am going to remove my child/children from the car," (clear communication) *and do it*. Don't get out of the car and walk back to open the rear door. This might enable the carjacker to shove you away, get behind the wheel, and drive off with your child still inside. Instead, stay in the car and climb over the seat to reach your child. If you have no choice and you must leave the car without your child, take the keys with you. Whatever you do, don't give a carjacker the opportunity to separate you from your child.

I recall hearing about one attempted carjacking where the woman said, "You're going to have to kill me because I am not going to let you drive off with my son." Although every situation is different, and no one response is the correct one, I remain full of admiration for her assertiveness and courage.

- **Getting stranded.**

   Late one night, a woman is driving alone. Her car gets a flat tire; she has to pull to the side of the highway. She knows it's dangerous to try and hitch a lift; at the same time, it seems equally dangerous to try and walk, or to wait inside her car. Then her worst fears are realized: she spots two men pulling up right behind her.

Or maybe the woman's car runs out of gas instead of breaking down, or she becomes stranded in a bad neighborhood instead of on the highway. There are countless versions of this woman-in-distress scenario, but they usually have these three things in common: *It's late, it's dark, and she's alone.*

If this kind of situation holds special fear for you, your anxiety might not be based solely on the real risks involved. You might also have been *conditioned* to be afraid. After all, how many times has someone told you (simply because you're a woman), "You shouldn't drive at night," or "You shouldn't travel alone"? How many times have you seen a movie in which the woman's car breaks down in one scene, and she's raped, assaulted, or killed in the next? This kind of conditioning only exacerbates a woman's valid fears of being stranded. It can have her believing, consciously or unconsciously, in the idea of the "helpless female."

Fortunately, there are specific things that you can do if you're ever stranded, and precautions you can take to avoid this situation altogether. I will describe these later and in depth in the chapter, "The Safety Factor: Your Personal Daily Checklist."

- **Being tied up or handcuffed.** This is something that I actually *want* you to be afraid of. Once you're tied up or handcuffed, your self-defense options drop to practically zero. You can try negotiation and other verbal techniques as a last resort, but there's no escaping the fact that you're completely at your attacker's mercy. And the rapist or attacker who ties his victim up means business: he usually does it so he can rape, torture, or murder his victim and take whatever time he needs to do so.

Speaking for myself, I would do just about anything to avoid being restrained in this way, and that includes risking a knife or gunshot wound. Don't ever buy into an aggressor's promise that he's not going to hurt you, that's he's "only" going to tie you up. If he pulls out a rope or a set of handcuffs, I strongly urge you to fight back with everything you've got.

10

DOMESTIC ABUSE

* Nearly one-third of all emergency room visits by women are attributed to domestic violence. *(American Medical Association)*
* Domestic violence is the number one cause of injury to women, more than auto accidents and muggings combined. *(American Medical Association)*
* Approximately one-third of all female homicide victims are killed by their husbands or boyfriends. *(FBI Uniform Crime Report)*

Perhaps you've heard these kinds of statistics before; you may agree that domestic abuse is a serious, widespread problem. Yet you might also be feeling that this subject has little if any direct bearing upon your life. Unless you're a so-called battered woman—for whom this chapter has painful and obvious relevance—you might be tempted to skip reading it entirely.

I urge you not to, however, and for many reasons. You may be suffering abuse without realizing that it *is* abuse. You might be in a relationship in which the warning signs that your partner will turn violent are subtle and easy to miss. You might have a friend or family member who is being abused and needs your help. Domestic abuse doesn't just occur in varying degrees, but takes many different forms. It can be verbal or psychological. It's not always as obvious as a punch in the face.

Invisible Wounds: The Legacy of Verbal Abuse

All domestic abuse begins with verbal abuse. But even if verbal abuse never escalates into physical violence, it is still abuse. While it doesn't leave bruises or black eyes, it can inflict just as much suffering on the victim, and take just as long to recover from.

The verbally abused woman often finds herself feeling isolated and confused. In her excellent book, *The Verbally Abusive Relationship,* author Patricia Evans notes that, "Friends and family may see the abuser as a really nice guy and, certainly, he sees himself as one." After all, he may argue, "I've never laid a hand on you." Nearly all verbal abusers deny that they are being abusive. They say, "You're making a big deal out of nothing," or "You're just too sensitive," or "I don't know what you're talking about." As a result, the victim is left feeling off-balance, confused, unsure of her own perceptions. She may come to believe that the problem lies with her. So she tries to be more understanding. She tries to be less demanding, or asks less from the relationship. She tries to overlook the abuse, or she begs for it to stop. Yet verbal abuse only stops when *both* partners are willing to change.

The verbal abuser is usually not abusive all the time. He may say (and mean), "I love you," "I need you," or "I couldn't live without you." But when he becomes irritable or angry, he "kicks the cat" and uses his partner as a scapegoat. Or when disagreements pop up, he becomes unable or unwilling to discuss them. Instead, he uses verbal abuse to assert his dominance and control.

Verbal abuse usually starts small, escalating over time (days, weeks, even years) into actual physical violence. For example, it may initially take the form of subtle put-downs or insults. These gradually give way to more overt criticisms or threats. Then the abuser starts using his physicality to assert his dominance. He may begin stepping into his partner's personal space, for example, forcing her to step back or move aside. He starts throwing his weight around, so to speak. This escalates into "playful" pinches or slaps on the rear end, or "unintentional" nudges or shoves.

These minor assaults then escalate into serious physical abuse: slaps, punches, or worse.

Identifying Verbal Abuse

Have you ever been, or are you now, the target of verbal abuse? Bear in mind that it doesn't always come in the form of an angry outburst punctuated by insults or obscenities. There are many ways to be verbally abused. Ask yourself whether your partner does any of the following:

- He uses argument instead of discussion when conflicts arise. Instead of making statements that begin with "I think . . . ," "In my opinion . . . ," or "If you ask me . . . ," he says "You're wrong!" or "You're crazy!" or "You don't know what you're talking about!"
- Your partner invalidates your hurt or angry feelings with statements like, "You're just too sensitive," or "You blow everything out of proportion."
- Your partner blocks you from communicating your requests, desires, or opinions. He habitually refuses to listen to you or talk to you. He says, "There's nothing to talk about," or gives you the "silent treatment." He says, "You know what I mean!" or "Just drop it!" or "Who asked you?" or he just gets up and leaves the room.
- Your partner uses insults and criticisms yet disguises them as jokes. When you say, "I didn't think that was funny," he responds with, "Oh, you just can't take a joke," "Lighten up!" or "Where's your sense of humor?" Or he responds with sarcasm ("Well *excuuuse* me").
- Your partner calls you names ("idiot," "bitch," "fatso"), whether angrily or "sweetly."
- Your partner puts the blame on you for any conflict. When you raise a grievance with him, he responds with "You're pushing my buttons!", "You just want to pick a fight!", or "There's no pleasing you!"
- Your partner continually assesses you, saying "You know what your problem is?" or "You know what the trouble with

you is?", then follows his judgments with criticisms ("You're never satisfied" or "You're lazy/stupid/too emotional").

- Your partner indicates that what you say or do is of no importance. When you offer an opinion ("I think the Democrats will win"), show him something you've done ("I redecorated the bedroom"), or simply relate good news ("I got a promotion at work"), he responds with, "So what?" or "Big deal" or "Who are you trying to impress?"

- Your partner erodes your self-esteem or determination with statements like, "You'll never succeed," "You'll never learn," or "It's too hard for you to understand."

- Your partner tells you what he wants instead of asking you; he says "Do this," "Do that," "Get off the phone!", or "Get out of here!" Or he tells you what you can't do: "You're not using the car," or "You're not going out tonight." He may also accompany his orders ("Do what I tell you . . .") with threats (". . . or I'm gonna get angry").

- When you try to discuss something that happened earlier, your partner says he doesn't remember it. He responds with, "I never said/did that," "I have no idea what you're talking about," or "You're imagining things."

- Your partner's anger is irrational and unpredictable; you never know what's going to make him mad.

- Your partner uses his anger to intimidate and frighten you.

Most of us (men *and* women) have probably said or done some of the above at one time or another. As the saying goes, we're only human. But if your partner does so repeatedly or habitually, if his behavior has become a pattern, you are living with a verbal abuser.

In a relationship, the goals of the verbal abuser and those of his partner are not the same: while she hopes for equality and mutual respect, he seeks to dominate and control. He may do so overtly, or covertly. He may shout and yell, or never raise his voice. He may explode in anger, or use more subtle means to attack his partner's self-esteem. But whatever form it takes, all verbal abuse stems from feelings of hostility.

One final thought. Although I will continue to discuss verbal abuse in the context of the male-female relationship, it's important to remember that, like physical violence, verbal abuse can come from any person in your life. It may come from a man or a woman, from a family member, friend, or co-worker. If you are a lesbian, it can come from a female partner. Yet whoever it comes from, it should never be tolerated in any form.

Stopping Verbal Abuse

If your partner is verbally abusive at the beginning of your relationship—when most people tend to be on their best behavior—chances are that the abuse will only get worse with time. True, he may just be repeating some bad habits he learned (and got away with) in previous relationships; if so, taking prompt, assertive action may nip those habits in the bud. But if someone shows a need to control or dominate you, or needs to vent his anger on you, it usually indicates deeper problems. I'd strongly advise you to end the relationship sooner rather than later.

But perhaps you're married, or in a long-term relationship in which you've invested a lot of time and energy. Hilda is a 74-year-old woman who attended one of my seminars. She approached me afterwards to say that her 79-year-old husband had become verbally abusive: yelling at her, ordering her around, and giving her the silent treatment for days and even weeks on end. When I asked her how long he had been treating her this way, she answered, "Oh, about forty years." For a variety of reasons—her age being just one of them—divorce or separation simply wasn't an option for Hilda. Yet she no longer wanted to tolerate her husband's behavior. You yourself may be in a similar situation. You want to stop your partner's verbal abuse, but for one reason or another, you don't want to end the relationship and abandon ship just yet.

If this is the case, you still can and should take action. It's never too late to start, and the first thing to do is begin setting boundaries. Once you decide to set boundaries or limits, you forget about trying to understand your partner's motives. You stop justifying, explaining, or trying to figure out what *you* did wrong. Instead, you recognize that verbal abuse is inappropriate whatever the circumstances, and you call him on *every* offense the moment it occurs.

Let's say you're watching television at home one night when your husband storms into the room. He yells, "Goddammit! You washed my best shirt and ruined it! You're such an idiot!" How do you respond? Do you apologize, or promise to be more careful in the future? Absolutely not. In this situation, it *does not matter* whether you ruined his shirt or not; all that matters is that he delivered his message in a verbally abusive way. *So forget about the message and focus on the abuse.* Say "Stop it right now! If you want to say something to me, say it politely," or "Hold it right there! I won't tolerate you yelling at me." Whenever possible, avoid delivering ultimatums ("If you don't stop yelling, we're through!"), which are usually just a feeble form of manipulation. Instead, state your message as a fact: "I will not tolerate that from you," or "Your language is unacceptable to me."

Be prepared for the fact that your partner may continue to argue with you or escalate his abuse. If he yells back, "You *are* an idiot!" (for example), say "I see," "So you say," or "That's what *you* believe." Then disengage from the discussion. You may not be able to stop the abuse then and there, but you don't have to stay around to listen to it.

Learning how to disengage is crucial, because not everyone reacts passively to verbal abuse. Apologizing, cowering, or bursting into tears are common responses, but a woman may just as easily get angry and give the abuser tit for tat. When he yells at her, she yells back; when he insults her, she insults him back. She matches his facial expression, tone of voice, and argumentative words. What is more, she may believe that this is the appropriate thing for her to do. "After all," she's thinking, "I'm not acting like a doormat, playing the victim, or taking his treatment lying down: I'm giving it right back!" Yet without realizing it, she may be ensuring that the verbal abuse will not only continue, but escalate. However satisfying an angry response may feel in the heat of the moment, it isn't the solution.

Whether a woman gets angry or breaks into tears, she may be giving her partner precisely what he wants, because an emotional reaction confirms that his words have gotten to her in some way. By engaging, the woman is drawn into the abuser's agenda. He becomes abusive, she gets angry, there's a cooling-off period, and the next time a conflict arises, the pattern repeats itself. It's a vicious cycle.

Remember: it takes only one person to initiate verbal abuse, but it takes two to have an argument. The solution, therefore, is not to respond aggressively, but assertively. Communicate that you will not tolerate another person's abuse, then disengage. "Leaving the arena" is not retreating; it's taking a step in the right direction.

I've met many women who left one verbally abusive relationship, only to suffer verbal abuse in the next relationship and the next. Yet far from being "unlucky in love," what they really lacked was an understanding of the patterns they were repeating. Fortunately, with the help of professional counseling and self-assessment, some of these women have been able to "break the cycle" and find lasting and healthy relationships.

Getting Help From Others

The verbally abused woman may initially turn to other people for support. Unfortunately, because most verbal abuse takes place with no one else around, friends or family members may react with skepticism ("Are you sure he really said that?") or downright disbelief ("I can't believe he'd say that"). So the victim begins to doubt her own perceptions and emotions.

Even when others react with sympathy, their well-meaning advice can carry a disempowering message:

- "You married him for better or worse." *(It's your responsibility to tolerate his abuse.)*
- "Men are like that sometimes." *(Learn to tolerate his behavior.)*
- "Don't expect so much." *(You don't deserve better treatment.)*
- "Try to be strong." *(You're feeling bad because you're weak.)*
- "Love conquers everything." *(If you become more loving, he'll stop being abusive.)*
- "All is fair in love and war." *(If you love him, you have to take his abuse.)*

- "It's not like he hit you or anything." *(Verbal abuse isn't really abuse.)*
- "Just keep on trying." *(It's up to YOU to fix the problem.)*
- "It takes two to have a problem." *(You're partly to blame.)*

Negative messages like these may also be offered to the woman who is being physically as well as verbally abused. Whatever the case, they do far more harm than good. The victim must ultimately turn to the only person who can really help her: herself. She must hold on to that part of her that says, "I am *not* imagining this. I am *not* to blame. I *do* deserve better treatment."

If you believe that you are a victim of verbal abuse, professional counseling can help you to understand and cope with it. If your partner refuses to attend counseling with you, go alone. Read all that you can about the subject; many books focus exclusively on verbal abuse and discuss it in far greater depth than I can hope to here. And never, ever forget that you can leave an abusive partner. You always have that choice, as difficult as it may be.

Physical Abuse: The Ultimate Betrayal

Identifying the Potential Batterer

Verbal abuse is a real indicator that your partner may one day use physical violence against you. However, it's not the only warning sign. Here are some others to watch for.

1. Your partner has a history of abuse. And that means abuse in *any* form. As statistics show, you are at risk if your partner has threatened, verbally abused, or physically abused other women in his life, such as an ex-wife or former girlfriend.

2. Your partner threatens you with violence. And that means *any* violence. Maybe he's never threatened to punch you in the mouth or break your neck. But has he ever raised his fist in anger? Has he ever said, "You're asking for it!" or "Do what I tell you, or I won't be responsible for my actions!"?

3. Your partner has hurt you. Has he ever shoved you, hit you, restrained you against your will, or grabbed you so hard it hurt? Even if he's only done it once—and promised that "it will never happen again"—the chances are that it will happen again and escalate further unless you take assertive action.

4. Your partner is controlling. All abuse—physical, verbal, and psychological—comes from a desire to dominate and control, and potential batterers generally have controlling and domineering personalities. Does your partner stop you from going out or seeing your friends? Does he stop you from using the family car or make you completely dependent on him for money? Does he tell you what you can or cannot wear? These are just some examples of controlling behavior.

Domestic violence rarely comes out of nowhere; men usually don't become batterers overnight. Physical abuse is always preceded by verbal abuse, and verbal abuse is usually preceded by controlling behavior.

Finally, other warning signs of a potential batterer to look for are negative or hostile attitudes towards women in general, excessive use of alcohol or drugs, and psychological or physical abuse during childhood at the hands of a parent or stepparent.

"The First Offense"

Some people might say that the best way to protect yourself from domestic abuse is to select the right partner in the first place. If only it were that easy. Even in an otherwise good marriage or healthy relationship, your partner may one day slip up and do or say something that you perceive to be abusive. Perhaps you're both running late for a party and he gives you a shove towards the door. Perhaps he uses abusive language. Maybe he grabs you in the heat of an argument, or throws some object in your direction.

What next? Do you file for divorce or otherwise call it quits? Is it inevitable that his actions will escalate into more serious abuse? In other words, are you at risk? There's only one way to find out: respond assertively right then, right there. Don't rationalize, excuse, or ignore his behavior. Protect your boundaries: make it clear in no uncertain terms that you find his behavior unacceptable and will not tolerate it. *And see how he responds*. Does he acknowledge that he was out of line, or does he try to justify his actions? Is he genuinely apologetic, or just telling you what he thinks you want to hear? Does he take you seriously, or tell you you're "overreacting"? More importantly, does he modify his behavior the next time you disagree?

We're treading on dangerous ground here because apologizing is one part of the cycle of abuse. The man who batters his partner nearly always apologizes later, and often very convincingly. He buys her flowers or some other kind of gift. He promises that it will never happen again. And yet at some point in the future it does happen again, and the cycle once again repeats itself.

For now, however, I'm focusing on what might be termed the "first offense"; namely, that initial, first-time abusive word or action that may occur in any relationship. If you take assertive action and your partner responds appropriately, you may opt to give him a second chance. But if the abuse ever reoccurs—and especially if it escalates—take it as a warning that it's time to rethink the relationship. It doesn't matter how long you've been married or living together, or how many kids you have, or how financially or emotionally dependent you may be on your partner: abusive behavior of any kind is unacceptable.

Common Misconceptions

Although many of the facts about domestic violence are becoming more and more familiar to the general public, myths and misinformation about the subject often take the place of truth.

Myth: Some women "just ask for it."

The truth is that no one deserves to be beaten, no matter what she says or does.

Myth: Wife-beaters are poor and/or uneducated.

Contrary to popular belief, domestic violence cuts across all socioeconomic lines. An abuser can just as easily be a wealthy, successful professional.

Myth: The only reason a woman stays with an abuser is because she doesn't have enough money to leave.

Financial dependence is only one of many reasons why a woman stays in an abusive relationship. Fearing retaliation, she may be too afraid to leave. She may be overwhelmed by feelings of guilt and shame. Over time, the abuse may have eroded her confidence and self-esteem to the point where she has lost all hope and even the will to live; this is known as Battered Women's Syndrome, and also includes such psychological disturbances as eating disorders, alcoholism, paranoia, and clinical depression.

Myth: Domestic violence is completely unpredictable.

In fact, domestic violence follows a recognizable cycle. It begins with a buildup of tension that may last days, weeks, or months. This tension eventually erupts into violence. The violence is followed by a period of tranquility; the abuser is contrite and apologetic. Then the cycle begins again.

Myth: Domestic violence means bruises or black eyes.

In other words, most abusers "only" slap their partners around. In reality, domestic violence can result in hospitalization and even death.

Domestic abuse also affects the entire family. Children who live in an abusive household are victims, too. They are at real risk of being battered themselves, and even if they only witness abuse, they suffer psychological damage. They're also more likely to grow up to become batterers and victims themselves than children who aren't in abusive families.

The Safety Hatch

Throughout this book, I have emphasized that your primary goal in the event of rape or assault should be to get to safety as soon as possible. This is a fairly straightforward concept when it applies to an attack on the street. If the attack comes from her husband or live-in partner, however, the woman who runs for safety may be fleeing the only home she knows. She may be leaving behind her money, possessions, even her children. For many women, this is paying too high a price for safety. And yet, staying where they are and suffering more abuse is equally unacceptable.

This is why I advise any woman who has been a victim of domestic abuse—and that means any abuse, at any point in the relationship—to plan ahead for her safety. First, pick a room in your home as a designated "safe room"; ideally, it should have a door with a strong lock, a window leading to the outside, and a phone. Second, hide an amount of cash in some secondary yet accessible location: in your car, for example (if you have your own), or even buried in your front yard. At the minimum, it should be enough to pay for taxi fare, phone calls, meals, and a hotel room for the night. Finally, hide an extra address book or list of phone numbers so you can contact a friend or family member in an emergency.

Preparation can be this simple or more elaborate. I had one student who xeroxed all joint financial statements; she felt this was information she would need "on the outside." Yet another student described one precaution she *wished* she'd taken. After she left an abusive husband, he methodically destroyed all her family photos and mementoes. These were her most treasured possessions, and in hindsight she wished she'd done something to protect them.

When people label these kinds of measures paranoid or extreme, they miss the point. Even if you never need to use your "safety hatch," just knowing that you have it can give you a feeling of confidence and peace of mind. It can foster a sense of independence rather than dependence. It can help you adopt a position of "zero tolerance" towards any form of domestic abuse.

Domestic Violence and Self-Defense

A woman is undressing for bed. Suddenly, a man enters the room and grabs her by the throat. He wrestles her to the floor and punches her in the face.

What should she do? From a purely self-defense standpoint, the answer is obvious: she should defend herself any way she can. She should fight with 100 percent commitment, causing whatever pain and injury she must in order to get to safety.

But let's suppose that her attacker is not an intruder, but her *husband.* Should her response be any different? Answer: NO! I don't care what your relationship is to your attacker—whether he's your husband, boyfriend, or a complete stranger—you still have the right to defend yourself. No one should have to endure pain and injury at the hands of another person, whatever the circumstances. Unfortunately, many victims of domestic violence do just that, and for many different reasons. A woman's self-confidence can be so eroded by past abuse, she becomes incapable of summoning the determination and commitment necessary to defend herself effectively. She may be paralyzed by shame or the fear of retribution, or she may simply not know how to fight. But more than anything else, it's usually the fact that a woman knows and possibly loves her attacker that stops her from defending herself effectively. It's always harder to defend yourself against someone you know. A woman may have shared a long history with her partner. She may have experienced happy times. He may be the father of her children. Unfortunately, the "ties that bind" can compromise her very instincts for survival.

A word of caution: if you do make the choice to defend yourself physically, I believe that you have to make it count. Slapping your abuser's face, for example, or throwing things in his direction, will only escalate the situation and place you at greater risk. By contrast, a well-placed attention-getter or forceful knee to the groin can disable him enough for you to get away.

Many women are reluctant to defend themselves effectively for fear of the legal repercussions. After all, they argue, it's one thing to drive your thumb into the eye of a rapist, another to do the same thing to the man you live with. I understand their concern; many women *have* gone to jail for retaliating against abusive partners. In nearly all such cases, however, the level of retaliation was disproportionately severe compared to the level of abuse. If your partner has been beating you, in other words, you don't have the right to kill him. If he has shoved you or slapped you, you don't have the right to blind him. But you *do* have the right to fight back in order to get to safety. I emphasize those words because you should never fight in order to exact retribution, get revenge, or "give him a taste of his own medicine." Whether you choose to defend yourself from your husband or a stranger, and whether you're on the street or in your home, you should fight for one reason only: to protect yourself, and get to safety.

When it comes to rape and assault on the street, planning ahead and living smart—rather than knowing how to fight—still remain your best defense. It's no different when it comes to domestic abuse. While every woman should know how to physically defend herself from an abusive partner, things should ideally never reach that stage. I had one student approach me and confide, "I'm in a physically abusive relationship, I need to know how to fight back." I helped her understand that physical retaliation wasn't her only option, or even the best one. We explored alternative techniques, such as verbal assertiveness, and focused on larger issues such as her own self-esteem. At the same time, I urged her to seek counseling, and to get out of the relationship entirely.

Domestic violence is as much a mental, emotional, and psychological threat as a physical one. If you have been a victim of chronic abuse, therefore, by all means learn the techniques of self-defense; they can empower you emotionally as well as physically. But don't stop there. Meet with anyone who can help you: therapist, counselor, lawyer. You need mental and emotional support far more than you need training in self-defense.

Safety Guidelines for the Battered Woman

If you are now a victim of physical abuse, the following guidelines can help protect you and your children while you seek further assistance.

1. Be prepared for a confrontation. Teach your children what they should do in the event of an emergency. Teach them how to dial 911, and how to get safely out of the house. Tell them where to go once they get outside (e.g. to a next-door neighbor to phone the police).

2. As soon as possible, report any incidence of physical battering to the police. Battering is not "a private matter." It's a criminal act, and calling attention to it can be your best protection. Remember: the police cannot protect you unless they know about the abuse. Just as importantly, there's a good chance that your batterer will not be prosecuted if you refuse to press charges.

Be prepared for the fact that not all police officers are trained to deal with domestic violence. Unless you *insist* on it, the officers who arrive at your home may not choose to make an arrest, especially if there is little physical evidence of assault (bruises, black eyes, etc.). If the police will not take your batterer into immediate custody, ask them to take you and your children to a safe place. At the same time, gather evidence you can later present to higher authorities. Write down the officers' names and badge numbers. If you receive medical treatment, obtain copies of your medical records and bills. Finally, ask someone to photograph your injuries as soon as possible.

It can be tremendously difficult for a woman to press charges against her partner. She may feel too guilty to do so. After all, this is someone she loves, and after an explosion of violence, her abuser will probably be contrite, apologetic, and even tearful. A woman may also hesitate to press charges because she is simply afraid to: she believes that her husband will retaliate as soon as he is released. Nevertheless, pressing charges is crucial if she wants to protect herself and her children. First, by bringing the problem out into the open it gives others the opportunity to help her. Second, it's a significant movement towards personal empowerment and away from victimhood. It's taking an all-important step in the right direction.

3. Exercise caution when preparing to leave an abusive relationship. All abusive relationships are based on a need for dominance and control. So when a woman takes control and tries to end the relationship, it can sometimes act as a trigger, causing her partner to become more violent.

The possibility of this occurring is a real one. So while your fear of retribution should never make you stay in an abusive relationship, you must exercise a particular degree of caution. In an assault situation, you should never run for safety unless you know that you can reach it; in a domestic violence situation, you should not attempt to leave before taking some important precautions:

- Make prior arrangements to stay with a trusted friend or loved one, at a location *unknown* to your partner.
- Have a bag packed with personal items you will need (car keys, phone numbers, identification). Obtain phone numbers of women's shelters and abuse hotlines.
- Learn about your legal rights. Contact the offices of your local prosecutor, attorney general, bar association, or battered women's shelter. If you can't afford an attorney, there are still ways to obtain an attorney's services at a reduced cost or at no cost to you at all.
- Get an Order of Protection. This is commonly known as a restraining order, and can provide you with legal protection from your batterer (or indeed, from a stalker, attacker, or harasser). With or without the help of a lawyer, you can obtain a restraining order from your local courthouse. Issued by a judge, it can order your batterer to stop physically or verbally abusing you or your children.

  In some circumstances, a restraining order can order your batterer to move out of your home, and to stay away from you, your family, your place of business, and your children's school. It can also give you custody of your children, and demand that your batterer seek counseling. In addition, some police departments will issue a short-term, emergency restraining order when officers visit the scene of a battering incident.

- Understand the limits of a restraining order. Be prepared for the fact that your partner may defy one. (While under the "protection" of an Order of Protection, a number of women have been tracked down and killed by their abusers.) Continue to exercise caution and your own intuition, awareness, and common sense.
- If you fear for your life and decide to carry a gun, learn how to use it. Just as importantly, understand that possession of a lethal weapon carries tremendous responsibilities,

including a legal one. I recall one case where an abused woman fled to a friend's home with her children; defying a restraining order, her partner tracked her down and broke into the house. Believing that he intended to kill her with his bare hands, the woman shot him dead, only to be tried and convicted for murder.

- Don't try to "go it alone." Physically exiting the house is only the first step towards understanding, preventing, and recovering from domestic violence. It's not just a safety issue, but one with tremendous legal, financial, and psychological implications, so take advantage of any and all outside resources that are available to you. One particular resource I highly recommend is the National Domestic Violence Hotline (1–800–799-SAFE); see *Resources* for more information on this service.

Domestic violence is an incredibly complex issue which I have really only touched upon in these few pages. Under *Recommended Reading,* you will find several excellent books which address the subject in the depth that it deserves. I strongly urge you to read at least one of them.

In order to close this section on a positive note, I'd like to share with you a letter I received from a woman after she attended one of my seminars. Her experience is a testament to the fact that however difficult it may be to do so, it *is* possible to escape the destructiveness of an abusive relationship.

Dear Mr. Marrewa: I am newly divorced and was in a very abusive relationship. The one thing I remember you talking about was intuition. My intuition when I first met my ex-husband was that he was not good for me. I let my reasoning and love override my gut feelings and I have suffered from the consequences. However, I have been in therapy and I have used my time to find out what I am about and to learn to love and accept myself again and not to blame myself. I wish you the best and maybe someday I will see you again.

11

RAPE: A CLOSER LOOK

You might say that we've been discussing rape throughout this entire book. From verbal empowerment to vital-target attacks, *everything* you've learned will help to protect you from a rapist.

Even so, I believe that the subject of rape merits an even closer look. First, because outside of domestic abuse, rape is the single most common form of physical assault against women. Second, because rape is in many ways unique. It differs from all other forms of assault for the following reasons:

- The causes, trauma, and repercussions of rape continue to be widely misunderstood by both men *and* women.
- The primary goal of the rapist is entirely different from that of the mugger, burglar, purse-snatcher, or carjacker.
- In contrast to other types of attackers, rapists often know their victims.
- Rape can occur on a date, or in the context of a boyfriend/girlfriend or husband/wife relationship.
- Rape is one form of assault that may leave no visible signs of injury. In its aftermath, therefore, special steps must be taken to preserve physical evidence that may implicate the rapist.

Rape doesn't happen to a faceless woman on the street, but to someone's mother, sister, daughter, wife, or friend. I know: I've seen their faces. To this day, I cannot remember facilitating a workshop where there wasn't at least one woman who had been raped. Chances are, you yourself know someone who has been raped, although you may not realize it: even today, the trauma and *stigma* of rape stops many women from reporting it, discussing it, or even acknowledging it.

Myth versus Truth: Understanding the Realities of Rape

Separating fact from fiction is vital to understanding the crime of rape. As with domestic abuse, myths about rape abound. The following provides a brief look at some of the more commonly held myths to date.

Myth: "Rape" means "sexual intercourse."
Rape includes other types of sexual assault. If a woman is sodomized, forced to perform oral copulation, or penetrated by a foreign object, she has been raped, even if sexual intercourse never took place.

Myth: Rape is about sex.
Rape is a crime of *violence* that is acted out sexually. The goal of the rapist is to dominate and degrade his victim; sex is only the vehicle by which he does this.

Myth: Most rapists are strangers to their victims.
A woman is *less* likely to be raped by a stranger than by someone she already knows: a friend, acquaintance, relative, neighbor, coworker, boyfriend, or husband.

When I ask my students to visualize a rapist, they usually describe a madman leaping from a darkened alley. Yet this scenario is the exception rather than the rule. Consistent with statistics, most of the rape survivors I've met knew their rapist.

Myth: Only young, attractive women are raped.
This myth stems from the misconception that rape is essentially a sexual act. It also contributes to another myth: that the woman

who dresses provocatively (short skirt, low-cut blouse, etc.) will be partly to blame if she is raped.

Rapists target *vulnerable* women, regardless of their age, appearance, race, religion, or physical description.

Myth: Rapes are usually unplanned. They most often occur late at night and away from home.
The vast majority of rapes are planned, occur during daylight hours, and occur inside or close to the victim's home.

Myth: Deep down, women *want* to be raped.
This has to be *one* of the most heinous myths perpetuated against women, but it just refuses to die.

A woman may want her sexual partner to be the "aggressor," and she may even enjoy "rough" sex, but this *doesn't* mean that she would enjoy being raped. In rape, the element of choice is missing altogether.

Ironically, some women have used this myth to their advantage in assault situations. By appearing to welcome the idea of sexual intercourse, they've lured their attackers into a false sense of security:

> *Renata was pinned down by a rapist in the back seat of her car. As he struggled to peel off her tight jeans, she cooed, "Here, maybe I can help you," and took them off herself. As if reassured, her attacker let his guard down for a moment, giving her just the opportunity she needed to inflict serious pain. She escaped this rape attempt with nothing but a few minor bruises. Her rapist ended up in the emergency room and then in prison.*

Myth: Rapists *look* like criminals.
A rapist can be dirty and unkempt, or handsome and well-dressed. He can be tall and muscular, or short and slightly built. He can be of any age, race, occupation, or physical description. *He can look like anyone.*

Myth: It's impossible to rape a non-consenting adult.
The mere *threat* of violence can immobilize anyone, especially if the rapist has a weapon. To break down her initial resistance, a

rapist may also slap, punch, or choke his victim, or inflict even more serious pain and injury.

Myth: To avoid injury, a woman should allow herself to be raped.

Rape is *itself* a traumatic injury. The woman who is raped but not otherwise injured has still been physically assaulted. She may bear emotional and psychological scars that can last a lifetime.

Myth: When it comes to rape, nonresistance is always the safest option.

Nonresistance is sometimes the *worst* possible option, especially if the rapist tries to tie up or handcuff his victim, force her into a car, or move her to a secondary location. Rape can be a prelude to torture, kidnapping, and murder; a woman can never be sure that her attacker "only" intends to rape her. In many situations, going on the offensive and counterattacking are far safer options than nonresistance.

The Mind of a Rapist

All attackers have two things in common: they select the most vulnerable and unsuspecting targets, and they use violence or the threat of violence to control their victims. Yet however dangerous a mugger or carjacker may be, his focus is not so much on you as on your purse, wallet, jewelry, or car. In other words, his primary goal is theft.

The rapist's goal is very different. He doesn't want a woman's possessions: he wants her body, her mind, her very soul. He wants to overpower, control, dominate, and violate her. Most rapists exhibit some degree of insecurity and self-centeredness in their behavior. They may use rape to compensate for the powerlessness they experience in daily life, or to give them an outlet for their inner frustration and rage.

Generally speaking, rapists fall into one of three categories: Stranger Rapists, Acquaintance Rapists, and Date Rapists. Keep in mind, however, that no matter who the rapist is or how well he knows his victim, *he is still a rapist.*

The **Stranger Rapist** may exploit a particular setting, such as an isolated jogging trail or a highway rest stop, and wait for the right victim to come along. But he may also use personal information, such as a woman's home address or her workplace hours, to select a time and place where she will be alone and most vulnerable. He may also use some ruse, whether simple or elaborate, to get inside a woman's home, car, or workplace.

You can be certain that this type of rapist has raped before. He's perfected his methods through experience. That's why reactions like crying, pleading, or backing away will not deter him from his attack. They're just what he expects; he's seen every one of them before. However, you can turn the tables on the stranger rapist by reacting in ways that he doesn't expect. These include calling, yelling, going on the offensive, and using the physical techniques of street fighting.

Studies have determined that **Acquaintance Rape** accounts for at least 60 percent of all rapes. Like stranger rapists, acquaintance rapists are opportunistic. However, while some date and stranger rapes can occur "spontaneously," with no prior plan or intention, the acquaintance rapist nearly always sizes you up ahead of time. With trust as his weapon of choice, he exploits the relationship that exists between you. He will test your boundaries, looking for signs of weakness and vulnerability. He will plan his attack, sometimes monitoring your movements for days, weeks, months, and even years.

A subcategory of acquaintance rape, **Date Rape** refers to attacks perpetrated by a man while on a date, or in the context of a "romantic" relationship (boyfriend, lover, etc.). I distinguish the date rapist from other types of rapists because he often has no prior intention to rape. (One exception to this is the date rapist who deliberately plies a woman with alcohol or drugs, then makes his move.) The date rapist may feel that he's "entitled" to sex with his date, especially if he has paid for the evening's entertainment. If his advances are rebuffed, therefore, he may take by force something he feels that he deserves. The date rapist may also force sex on a woman because he believes that, deep down, it's what she really wants; in his mind, "no" means "yes." Very often, this kind of date rapist doesn't see himself as a rapist.

The date rapist is arrogant, self-centered, and a bully. He seldom uses a knife or gun. Instead, trust, intimidation, manipulation, and physical force (or just the threat of physical force) are *his* weapons of choice.

Your "Achilles' Heel"

Physically defending yourself from any rapist is daunting, but it becomes even more so if you already know your rapist. Many people can picture themselves going all-out to defend themselves from a stranger, but cannot visualize inflicting the same pain and damage on a co-worker, classmate, or neighbor. Their visualization becomes harder still if the aggressor is their "friend," relative, boyfriend, or husband.

As a general rule, I believe that the more intimate you are with your rapist, the harder it is to defend yourself. What's worse, the acquaintance rapist or date rapist *knows* this. He takes this Achilles' heel and exploits it to his advantage. For that reason, it's essential that you understand and believe one very important thing: once someone you know crosses the line into attempted rape, he becomes *no different* than a stranger rapist, and the rape that occurs on a date or in the context of a romantic relationship is *no different* than the rape that occurs in a darkened alley, deserted park, or underground parking garage.

Advantage: You

When it comes to a rapist, you can never judge a book by its cover; appearances really can be deceiving. Yet very often, this is one axiom that the rapist himself forgets. Even as he assesses his victim's weaknesses, he may underestimate her real strengths. That's *his* weakness, and you can use it to your advantage.

> *A rapist spotted Denise exiting a market and targeted her for attack. She looked like an easy score: she's small and petite, she's in her 50s, and she was walking alone. Her car was a good distance away; the parking structure was dimly lit. The rapist assumed that he had this one in the bag.*

In fact, this rapist seriously underestimated his intended victim. Despite her age, build, and deceptively frail appearance, Denise is actually tough-minded, physically trained, and was prepared to fight back. When the rapist made his move, therefore, he got far more than he bargained for. He suddenly found himself on the defensive. He learned that his size and strength were no protection from effective self-defense techniques and total commitment on her part.

And here's an important point: Denise took her rapist by surprise not so much by resisting, but by resisting in ways he didn't predict. Her attacker expected Denise to scream, plead for mercy, or try to run away, perhaps, or to fight defensively by clawing, kicking, shoving, or struggling to break free. He *didn't* expect her to deliberately get close, fight offensively, and inflict serious pain and damage.

It's a fact that most people know nothing about self-defense, and this can be used to your advantage. The techniques you have learned are effective in and of themselves, but are doubly effective because they can take your rapist by surprise. The chances are overwhelmingly in your favor that he has *never encountered them before*.

The Aftermath of Rape

In the minutes following a sexual assault, decision-making of any kind can be overwhelming. That's why I believe every woman should know *ahead of time* what to do in the event that she is raped. These steps will not only help to protect her, but may help bring her rapist to justice.

Get to safety as soon as possible. Before you even try to phone for help, get to a safe location. Some rapists return to the scene of the crime to rape their victim a second time.

Call a trusted friend or loved one. You are going to need someone to lean on as you meet with police, undergo a medical examination, and deal with the psychological aftermath of rape.

The person you call may not necessarily be your husband or closest family member. You must have someone with you who is not only supportive and nonjudgmental, but emotionally strong. A spouse or family member may be too upset by your rape to remain objective or offer real support. You may end up having to calm and comfort him or her at a time when you should be focusing on your own emotions.

If you don't have a friend or relative to call, you can contact a sexual assault center in your area. They will send out a volunteer to be with you, possibly a woman who has been raped herself and can relate to your experience. In addition, many police departments and hospitals employ rape crisis counselors who can offer you specialized support.

Don't do anything to disturb the crime scene. You don't want to destroy any physical evidence (semen, saliva, blood, hair samples, fibers, fingerprints, etc.) that might be used to implicate your rapist.

For the same reason, resist the natural urge to bathe or take a shower. Don't even wash your hands, brush your hair, or change your clothing. If you really have to change your clothes, put them in a paper bag (plastic destroys some types of evidence) and take them with you to the hospital or police station. If you have to urinate, do so in a jar; otherwise, important evidence may be lost.

Report the rape to police. Do this no matter who has raped you: stranger, friend, acquaintance, date, relative, boyfriend, or husband. Rape is rape. Period.

Try to cooperate with the police as fully as you can. This can be harder than it sounds. You may be asked to repeat your story again and again, as though the police do not believe you. In fact, this is really the best way for them to determine the facts. You may be asked hundreds of questions, and many of them may seem bizarre ("Did he use a condom?"), intrusive ("Are you a virgin?"), and embarrassing ("Did penetration occur? Was it vaginal, rectal, or oral?"). Try to answer them fully; your answers may enable authorities to identify, apprehend, and prosecute your rapist.

The majority of rapes in this country are not reported to police, and for a variety of reasons. The rape survivor may be so traumatized, she feels she cannot face the added trauma of police questioning and medical examinations. She may be overwhelmed by feelings of shame and guilt. She may fear retaliation; after all, nearly all rapists threaten their victims with bodily harm or death, as in "If you tell anyone, I'll track you down and kill you." Finally, the rape survivor may fear that no one will believe her story, especially if she knows the rapist and bears no visible signs of injury, such as cuts or bruises.

There are many reasons, however, why it is important to report your rape to the police. The first and most obvious is that it could lead to your rapist being caught and convicted. Most rapists are repeat offenders, and are likely to rape again and again unless they are caught. By reporting your attack, therefore, you might just save other women from the same brutality. Yet reporting a rape has another, equally important benefit: it can be the first step towards regaining control over your life.

Seek medical attention as soon as possible. Do this even if you do nothing else. Go to the nearest emergency room, and tell the nurses and doctors that you have been raped. Seek medical attention even if you don't appear to be injured; you may have unknowingly suffered internal injuries, or you may be going into shock. Also, a prompt physical examination can make all the difference in retrieving important physical evidence.

Here's what to expect at the hospital. You'll have to answer some routine questions (your name, age, medical history), but also some more intrusive ones, such as what type of birth control you use or the date of your last period. You may be asked to give samples of your hair, including pubic hair. You may be asked to give a detailed description of the assault; this will help the doctor determine how and where you were hurt, and where to look for evidence.

You will be checked for visible injuries, then given a pelvic examination so the doctor can look for signs of recent intercourse (such as vaginal inflammation or the presence of semen). Finally, the doctor may address your concerns about pregnancy and sexually-transmitted diseases.

If you are capable of doing so, write down anything you can remember about the attack. Exactly how, when, and where did the assault occur? What did your rapist look like, how was he dressed, and what did he say to you? Record as many details as you can. One rape survivor could only remember that her rapist had "smelled bad," yet based on that seemingly insignificant clue, police focused their suspicions on a man in her neighborhood. Armed with a search warrant, they searched his apartment and found evidence that positively linked him to the crime.

Don't blame yourself for the rape. Don't fall into making "If only" or "I shouldn't have" statements, as in "If only I hadn't walked to my car alone," or "I shouldn't have been in that neighborhood." You are never to blame for an assault, no matter what you may have said or done.

Seek professional counseling. Feelings of fear, guilt, embarrassment, anger, and helplessness are all common to women who have endured the trauma of rape. It's vitally important that you contact a counselor to help you work through these feelings and set you on the road to recovery. A sympathetic, trained professional can make all the difference. Your local hospital, rape crisis center, or police department can help put you in touch with programs and counselors in your area.

Date Rape

Ask single women about the downside of being single, and dating is one word that seems to pop up with depressing frequency. Maybe it's because the woman entering today's singles scene has to contend with more than the usual "dates from hell" and blind dates that don't pan out. She must also adapt to changing gender roles and shifting attitudes about sexuality, and she must protect herself from sexually-transmitted diseases, especially HIV. And as if this weren't enough, she must be prepared to defend herself from date rape.

If you're already married or in a committed relationship, you might be feeling that date rape is something you no longer have to worry about. After all, the very term implies rape that occurs only during a casual date. Yet I've met many women who were "date-raped" by boyfriends with whom they had a steady, long-term relationship, or by men they worked or went to school with and considered to be friends. Whether you call it date rape or acquaintance rape, there are many reasons why *every* woman should understand why and how it occurs.

1. You have a daughter who is of dating age. Statistics show that teenage girls and college-age women are the most vulnerable to date rape.

2. You have single girlfriends who date. The woman who is knowledgeable about date rape can be a better friend to single girlfriends who may not be so well-informed.

3. Not all relationships last. You may be in a committed relationship now, but may one day return to the dating scene.

4. You don't have to be dating to be date-raped. An assault can occur during a seemingly innocent social encounter, such as a drink with a co-worker. It can also occur in the context of a long-term, committed relationship.

Blaming the Victim

Date rape *is* rape. But the woman who is raped in a social context, by a man she already knew and willingly consorted with, rarely receives the same level of understanding and sympathy as the woman assaulted by a stranger on the street. All too often, other people blame the victim as much as they do the rapist and may offer the "shouldn't have" response, as in:

"She shouldn't have invited him to her apartment."
"She shouldn't have had so much to drink."
"She shouldn't have led him on."
"She shouldn't have trusted him."
"She shouldn't have gotten into his car."
"She shouldn't have let him kiss/touch/fondle her."

In other words, they imply that she was totally or partly responsible for her own misfortune. Take the Mike Tyson/Desiree Washington rape case of some years back. Many people still believe that Washington had no business being in Tyson's hotel room at 2:00 a.m., that she was "just asking for it." Talk about a double standard. Imagine if an acquaintance invited me to have a beer at his apartment, and then beat me to a pulp. Would anyone say I "just asked for it" by going to his apartment, or that I had "only myself to blame"? Washington may have been naive, she may have used poor judgment, but she didn't deserve to be raped. No woman does, regardless of what she says or does, what she wears, or how much she has to drink.

In recent years, some people have extended the definition of date rape to include situations where a woman willingly sleeps with a man only to regret her decision the next day, or when a man uses lying, manipulation, or *any* form of pressure to obtain a woman's sexual favors. I believe that this mind-set does a great disservice to women who have suffered the serious trauma of rape. When I refer to rape, I'm referring to any type of *forced* sexual assault, whether it takes the form of sexual intercourse, sodomy, penetration with a foreign object, or oral copulation, and regardless of who carries it out, whether husband, boyfriend, casual date, friend, co-worker, or complete stranger.

Date Rape on Campus

When I was a member of a college fraternity in the late 1970s, a campus official stopped by to warn us about the risks of getting female students drunk with the aim of taking advantage of them. However, he wasn't concerned with the risks to the women themselves, but to *the fraternity members!* We were cautioned that if we engaged in sexual misconduct on our premises, we could be suspended, expelled, or—as had happened to other fraternities around the country—lose our charter to operate on campus. Not surprisingly, this official never used the term "rape"; he probably thought of rape as a crime committed by violent street thugs, never by clean-cut college boys.

One would like to believe that his brand of ignorance and sexism has disappeared for good. Unfortunately, date rape on campus is as rampant as it ever was. Wild parties, the abuse of alcohol and drugs, the sudden escape from parental authority, you name it: the very circumstances of campus life put the college woman at special risk.

Protecting Yourself from Date Rape

You will markedly decrease your chances of becoming a victim of date rape if you adhere to the following guidelines.

1. Play an active role in planning a first date. Would you give a perfect stranger your phone number and home address? Would you let him come inside your home? Would you ride with him in his car? Answer: not unless you had no choice. Yet when that stranger is a first date, it's downright traditional for a woman to do all these things and more.

Earlier, I urged you never to trust anyone blindly, and that principle is no less true when it applies to someone you're dating. Until you've gotten to know your escort, until he has earned your trust, always follow these simple precautions:

- Don't automatically give out your home telephone number. Instead, exercise your power and ask for *his* number, or provide your work number only.
- Don't initially give out your home address. Instead, arrange to meet at a public place where you feel comfortable. Drive to and from that place yourself so you're not dependent on your date for transportation.
- Ask questions. Learn as much as you can about a prospective date ahead of time. Whenever possible, talk to friends you have in common. At the very least, find out where he lives and where he works. Although there are no guarantees, common sense dictates that the more you know about some- one, the better.
- Let a friend or loved one know where you're going and with whom, and when you expect to return home.
- Never accept a ride or go home with someone you don't know.

2. Communicate clearly. Miscommunication is a contributing factor in many date rapes. Never assume that your date knows how intimate you do or do not want to get. Be as open and straightforward as possible, and back up your words with appropriate body language. For example, if you've just left a long-term relationship and you're not ready for another sexual relationship, say so. Speaking as a man, I can tell you that the only way your date will know where you're "coming from" is if you tell him.

3. Listen to your intuition. It's easy to get caught up in the excitement of a date, and perhaps only natural to feel a little nervous. But if your feelings ever cross the line into discomfort, uncertainty, or irritation, take the time to examine why. Is your date crossing your personal boundaries by getting too close physically, or by asking intrusive or inappropriate questions? All too often, we ignore our gut feelings because we want to make a good impression. But rape can happen to anyone, at any time and in any place, so use your inner voice as an "early warning system." If you start to feel uncomfortable or unsafe while on a date, just get up and *leave*. Never compromise your safety.

4. Set high standards. Expect to be treated with respect and dignity by anyone you date. Expect your wishes to be honored. If they aren't, end the date immediately.

5. Don't allow anyone to "buy" your affections. There are still plenty of men who feel that if they buy a woman gifts or treat her to an expensive dinner, they deserve something in return, whether that something is a kiss at the doorstep or an entire night in her bed. This type of man may become resentful and angry when his expectations are rebuffed; he may even get physically aggressive.

The only thing you "owe" a date is the pleasure of your company, and even that is given at your discretion. If he tries to make you feel obligated to bestow any sexual favor, take assertive action. Tell him he's out of line, and end the date right there. Some women get around this problem entirely by offering to pay their own way; this can be viewed as a courtesy and as a precaution.

6. Limit your consumption of alcohol. Anything that inhibits your ability to think clearly will increase your vulnerability to date rape.

A disturbing number of my students were victims of date rape when they were younger, even though they didn't realize at the time that it *was* rape. The majority of these attacks involved the use of alcohol. Chloe's story is typical. While her date refrained from drinking, he plied her with alcohol until she eventually passed out. When Chloe regained consciousness some time later, she was on the floor and he was sexually assaulting her. She remembers saying no, she remembers trying to push him off, and she remembers feeling ashamed the next day for her own "stupidity." Not until 20 years later did she understand that taking advantage of someone who is mentally or physically incapable of giving consent (as Chloe was when she was drunk) is rape. When Chloe did realize this, it was as though the attack had occurred just yesterday; she needed therapy to help her cope with her emotions.

If you choose to drink alcohol on a date, know your tolerance and set limits on how much you plan to drink. Try to surround yourself with a friend or friends with the understanding that you'll look out for one another. And watch how much alcohol your date is consuming. Many otherwise trustworthy people become abusive when under the influence.

7. Beware of "date rape drugs." Virtually odorless and color-less, these may be slipped into your drink without your knowledge. *Rohypnol* (often known on the street as "Roofies") is one of the most dangerous. Within 30 minutes of ingestion, it causes drowsi-ness, disorientation, impaired judgment, and blackouts, and its effects can last for several hours. What makes rohypnol particularly dangerous is that it also causes memory loss and temporary amne-sia; a woman may be raped while under its influence, then have little or no memory of the assault. To make matters even worse, rohypnol is inexpensive, sometimes sold for as little as $2–$4 per tablet. Yet another drug that has been linked to date rape is *gamma-hydroxybutyrate* (GHB), commonly referred to as "Liquid Ecstasy" for its alleged ability to increase sexual arousal and lower a person's inhibitions. Like rohypnol, GHB is colorless, with a mildly salty taste that is easily disguised when mixed into a drink.

The initial symptoms of GHB and rohypnol—slurred speech, loss of coordination, bloodshot eyes, disorientation—are such that the user appears to be extremely intoxicated; therefore, other people may simply assume that she's just had too much to drink. Unfortunately, the amnesiac qualities of these drugs (especially rohypnol) leave the user particularly vulnerable to date rape. Young women given these drugs without their knowledge have reported waking up in frat houses without their clothes on, on the street, or in unfamiliar surroundings with unfamiliar people.

As if date rape and unprotected sex weren't enough to worry about, rohypnol and GHB can also cause respiratory distress, coma, and even death. In one documented case, for example, a 17-year-old woman who unknowingly ingested GHB that had been slipped into her soft drink later died from its effects.

To ensure that this never happens to you, only consume a beverage if you know what it contains and where it came from. Don't accept a taste of someone else's drink. Try to watch as your drink is being prepared, and accept it only from a waiter or bartender. Never leave your drink unattended or drink anything, such as mixed punch, if you are unsure of its ingredients.

"Date Harassment"

A woman and her date arrive back at her apartment; she doesn't invite him in. In the time-honored tradition of the ardent male, he pressures her for a good-night kiss. She doesn't want him to kiss her, but she gives in; maybe it seems a small concession to get him out of her hair. Unfortunately, he takes her acquiescence as a green light to get even more physical. Before she knows it, she's locked in a wrestling match and it's all she can do to get inside and slam the door.

Sound familiar? It probably does. Society has almost come to accept this scene as a ritual of dating. It's been replayed countless times in movies and TV shows, and often for comic effect. But there's nothing funny about being cornered by a sexually aggressive date who uses his physicality to "extort" a good-night kiss (or more). At the very least, it can be obnoxious and irritating; at worst, it's intimidating and even threatening. It's also a form of harassment that is endemic; I've had hundreds of women ask me how they should deal with sexually aggressive dates. My answer is always the same: adopt an attitude of "zero tolerance" towards any date who tries to touch you, kiss you, or restrain you against your will.

Why do I sound so emphatic? Partly because it's a question of simple self-respect; no one, man or woman, should have to submit to a violation of their personal boundaries. But it's also a safety issue. The best way to protect yourself from date rape is to establish your personal boundaries early, and protect them assertively. It's easier to take control at the beginning of a date, and indeed, at the beginning of a relationship; the longer you wait, the harder it gets. So if you don't like something, whether it's an "innocent" arm around your shoulder or something more intrusive, put a stop to it right then and there.

Not all unwelcome advances are a prelude to date rape, of course (a man may be assertive or persistent without ever turning aggressive), and how you discourage an unwelcome advance is a matter of personal preference. Sometimes body language is all it takes: maybe a cold stare, a look down at the offending arm, or a simple move away will do the trick. But if your body language doesn't get your message across, don't hesitate to speak up. You can be blunt or you can be diplomatic, but whatever you do, make it clear what you do or do not want. And if your date still doesn't back off, *take that as an indicator.* The man who doesn't honor your boundaries when it comes to small things is showing you neither consideration nor respect; even worse, he may become the date *rapist* who won't take no for an answer. It happens all too often.

Many times, a woman refrains from speaking up because she fears it will ruin an otherwise lovely evening, or even the relationship itself. She may see boundary-setting as an all or nothing choice between keeping quiet and getting downright nasty. As I've said before, however, you can be assertive yet diplomatic, as in "I really like you, but I think it's too early for that," or "I've had a great time tonight, but I'm not ready to get physical." Or open with simple honesty: "I want to be straight with you" or "I want you to know how I feel." The dialogue is up to you, as long as you remember that while you can open with something tactful, positive, or downright flattering, you should always end with a definite statement. If your request is ignored, throw diplomacy to the winds and use verbal self-defense ("Back off!"). Never let the fear of making waves trap you into tolerating something unwelcome or inappropriate.

And if all your verbal methods fail, don't hesitate to employ some form of physical self-defense. In situations where someone just refuses to back off, a well-placed attention-getter can work wonders while not inflicting serious damage. A slap to the testicles, an ear box, an elbow to the ribs, a hammer strike to the nose, or any of the techniques to escape a grab or hold I described earlier should enable you to get to safety.

Reluctant to fight fire with fire and resort to physical techniques? Don't be. While it *is* harder to get tough with someone you know than with a stranger, don't allow that fact to turn you into a victim. If there's anything I want you to take from this chapter, it's the following: it doesn't matter who a man is. It doesn't matter if he's a boyfriend, acquaintance, or casual date. As soon as he uses his physicality to restrain you against your will, he becomes *no different* than some jerk trying to grope you on the subway. And in many ways, he's even worse: he's abusing the trust you've placed in him.

12
SPECIAL TOPICS

Ordinary People: The Everyday Victims of Stalking

Like sexual harassment, stalking existed well before it received a trendy label. The good news is that it has been publicized more in recent years, largely because of celebrities who have been stalked. Of these incidences, the murder of actress Rebecca Schaeffer—shot on her apartment doorstep by a delusional admirer—is perhaps the most notorious. Other celebrity targets of stalking have included actresses Jodie Foster and Teresa Saldana, tennis star Monica Seles, and U.S. Olympic skier Patricia Kastle. Kastle was stalked for months by her ex-husband, and had a restraining order in her purse when he eventually shot and killed her.

Yet despite the focus on celebrities, the vast majority of stalking victims are ordinary people. And while it's true that men are sometimes stalked—directly or indirectly (as when a stalker goes after his victim's new boyfriend)—the overwhelming majority of stalking victims are women, most of whom are stalked by men they already know.

Stalking can take a severe emotional toll on its victim, whether she is physically assaulted or not. It robs her of her freedom and security. Two particular factors make stalking so traumatic: its unpredictability, and its duration (many victims are stalked over a period of years). Because they live in a virtual state of siege, most stalking victims display stress-related symptoms, including backaches, headaches, sleeplessness, nightmares, ulcers, anxiety attacks, clinical depression, and Post-Traumatic Stress Disorder.

What is Stalking?

Stalking is, quite simply, *repeated* harassment or following. It has achieved some long-overdue legal recognition in recent years: California set a precedent in 1990 when it became the first state to pass anti-stalking legislation, and today, every state in the country has similar laws on their books. These laws may vary from state to state but generally define stalking as a willful, malicious and repeated pattern of harassment or following. The key words here are "repeated pattern," because more than one incident needs to take place before the behavior can be classified as stalking. If someone sends you one threatening letter, that's harassment. But if he sends you two, three, or four threatening letters, that's stalking because he has demonstrated a *pattern* of behavior.

In its early stages, stalking behavior can easily be mistaken for normal romantic interest. After all, things like telephoning, driving past someone's house, or sending romantic notes are not inappropriate in and of themselves. As a result, many victims do not recognize that a problem exists until the stalking becomes more threatening.

That's why it's important for you to understand the many forms of stalking. If someone does any of the following things *repetitively,* then it constitutes stalking behavior:

- **Harasses you by phone:** calls and hangs up, or remains silent; phones repeatedly, or leaves disturbing or threatening messages
- **Sends letters or cassette tapes:** these may be rambling, obscene, or threatening
- **Sends unwanted gifts**
- **Approaches people in your life:** to deliver threats, or to get personal information about you
- **Follows you:** either by car or on foot

- **"Shadows" you:** cruises past your home or workplace
- **Turns up uninvited:** where you live, for example, or where you work, exercise, dine out, or go to school
- **Keeps you under "surveillance":** waits outside your home, for example, or spies on you through your windows
- **Threatens you with erratic or "crazy" behavior**
- **Vandalizes your property:** slashes your car tires, for example, or breaks your windows, sprays graffiti across your property, or harms your pet
- **Commits theft:** steals anything—however small—from your home, office, car, or yard

Even more serious stalking behaviors include trespassing, breaking and entering, physical assault (including rape and kidnapping), attempted murder, and murder.

Types of Stalkers

Not all stalkers are actually insane. Many suffer from personality disorders which fall well short of serious mental illness. Yet in one way or another, all stalkers display aberrant behavior.

By far the most common form of stalking in this country is **domestic violence stalking.** This is when an abusive ex-husband or former boyfriend stalks his former partner. Statistics show that the abusive ex-partner is a particularly dangerous type of stalker. He represents a triple threat: he knows his partner intimately, he has a track record of violence, and he is often determined to reassert control.

When a woman tries to leave an abusive partner—or indeed, makes *any* move towards independence—it can put her at added risk. The abuser may feel hurt, abandoned, and rejected, but these feelings manifest themselves as a desire for revenge. This type of stalker goes after his partner to "teach her a lesson" or to "show her who's boss." He cannot accept himself as the loser and his partner as the winner; he must restore the status quo. He is extremely possessive; he believes that he owns his partner. His attitude is often, "If I can't have you, nobody will."

Like domestic violence itself, domestic violence stalking usually follows a recognizable cycle. It begins with a gradual build-up of tension: the stalking escalates from annoying phone calls to surveillance, perhaps, or from surveillance to open threats. The tension then explodes into physical violence that may be directed towards the victim herself, towards her property or pet, or towards a relative or boyfriend. This may be followed by a deceptively calm phase in which the stalker asks for forgiveness or backs off. But it can also be followed by a final act of control: murder, suicide, or both.

The **casual acquaintance** stalker is someone you know: a co-worker, perhaps, or a client, landlord, or next-door neighbor. Or he may be someone you interact with regularly yet very superficially: a supermarket clerk, for example, or a fellow member at your gym.

This type of stalker perceives your relationship to be closer than it really is, or expects more from the relationship than you are willing to give. You may initially feel perplexed by his behavior; it may strike you as simply odd or inappropriate. Later, as the stalking escalates, his behavior starts to leave you feeling threatened or disturbed.

You may also be stalked by **someone you have dated.** When you try to break off the relationship, this type of stalker simply won't let go. He won't take no for an answer. He goes into a "candy and flowers" phase: phoning you repeatedly, sending you romantic cards, love notes, or unwanted gifts. You may initially be flattered by his behavior, because this type of stalker often portrays himself (and is seen by others) as a brokenhearted lover or lovesick admirer. Then his behavior escalates: the notes become more insistent, perhaps, or he begins to show up uninvited at your home or workplace. You may also be stalked by **someone you turn down for a date.** When you thwart his advances, he becomes hostile. His ego has been hurt, and he's looking for payback.

In rarer cases, a stalker may choose a **random target.** He meets her once or twice and develops a fixation. Still other victims are stalked **anonymously;** they never learn their stalker's identity.

Stalking in the Workplace

A stalker often targets his victim where she works, and for the most obvious of reasons: along with her home, it's one place where he knows she can be found. Also, because the workplace throws together people who might not otherwise associate, it's one place where harassment and then stalking can start.

If a woman is stalked by a co-worker, getting him fired rarely puts an end to the problem. Indeed, it may cause the stalking to take a more threatening turn. Women also have been fired from their jobs after their employers learned that they were being stalked. A boss may not want the aggravation, or may not want to put other employees at risk. He may also hold the woman partially to blame, especially if the stalker is her ex-husband or ex-boyfriend.

How to Protect Yourself from a Stalker

1. Listen to your intuition. The available data on stalkers confirms that most of them share certain traits. They're usually insecure, possessive, and controlling, so they have trouble sustaining normal friendships and relationships. They often pride themselves on their ability to deceive; they see themselves as being exempt from society's laws, social mores, and codes of behavior. They also have a low threshold for frustration, and a tendency to blame other people for their problems. Sometimes, traits like these are so obvious, they constitute a virtual "red flag." Yet in many situations, the signs are very subtle and easy to miss, or they may take many months to emerge; therefore, it can be hard to recognize or pinpoint when someone's behavior crosses the line from appropriate to inappropriate, from normal to abnormal. Quite often, a woman's only clue to a potential stalker may be the bad feeling or vibe she gets when he's around.

That's why it's so essential to trust your intuition. Before your mind recognizes that a problem exists, your intuition can put you on alert; it's the ultimate early-warning system. Therefore, do not wait until the stalking becomes overt. If someone's behavior seems suspicious, inappropriate, or abnormal, or if it simply makes you feel nervous, disturbed, or threatened, *take action.*

It's crucial to trust your intuition because while it may be telling you one thing, the other people in your life may be telling you another. Be warned: there are no guarantees that your friends, family, and co-workers will respond with support and understanding if you tell them that you are being stalked. Stalking is a widely misunderstood phenomena, and other people may minimize the problem, as in "It's just a phase." They may also interpret the stalker's behavior as normal, romantic persistence:

"Oh, he's just got a crush on you."
"You should be flattered."
"What did you expect? You're an attractive woman."

They may propose simplistic solutions:

"Just ignore him."
"Humor him."
"Have your husband/boyfriend/father set him straight."

They may imply that *you* are to blame:

"What did you say or do to set him off?"
"You're too nice to people."
"You shouldn't have been so friendly."
"You shouldn't have gone out with him in the first place."

Finally, they may react with skepticism or downright disbelief:

"You're imagining things."
"You're being paranoid."
"You're overreacting."
"You're making this up."

Or they may do all of the above. That's why it's so essential to trust your intuition. You are feeling and reacting in a particular way for a reason: your inner voice is telling you that your stalker's behavior *is* serious and illegal and *isn't* your fault. So listen to that voice: it's telling you the truth.

2. Set boundaries. With stalking, as with any form of harassment, setting boundaries should be your first line of defense. Setting boundaries is one way of empowering yourself, and in many cases, may be enough to stop the stalking in its tracks. So spell it out. As explicitly and clearly as possible, tell the person harassing you to stop the harassment immediately.

Many women hope to discourage a stalker by letting him down gently, but this gradual approach usually backfires. Rather than deterring a stalker, it is more likely to encourage him; he takes it as a sign that the victim cares for him and is sensitive to his feelings. Therefore, be direct and unequivocal. DO NOT WAIT to take action; stalking behavior rarely stops or tapers off on its own. And once you've clearly set your boundaries, do not engage in any further dialogue with the stalker: not in person, not by phone, not even through the mail. Any further communication should come through a third party, such as your attorney.

3. Document, Document, Document. As with other threats of violence, document the stalker's behavior. Taking a proactive approach can help to empower you in what may seem like an otherwise helpless situation. Collecting evidence is also crucial if you want to build a legal case. *You will not be able to implicate your stalker without evidence and documentation,* so start collecting it now.

- Keep a journal. Describe *every* contact and conversation that you have with the stalker: what he said and did, when and where the contact occurred, and the names of any witnesses. Taken individually, these incidents may seem insignificant; when amassed over a period of weeks or months, however, they will constitute a body of evidence against your stalker.
- Keep all cards, letters, cassette tapes, and gifts sent to you by the stalker.
- Keep all messages left on your answering machine or voice mail. If you are stalked by phone, you might be tempted to get an unlisted number or to disconnect your phone. Think twice before doing either one of these things! Answering machines can be used to collect evidence that may implicate your stalker. Also, if your stalker cannot reach you by phone, he may resort to more direct forms of communication: turning up at your workplace, for example, or con-

tacting your family or friends. So keep your phone line open, and your answering machine on at all times.

- Write down the license number, make, and model of your stalker's car.

- Try to photograph your stalker. You can make copies from a photograph and distribute them to people you know (so they know who to watch out for). A photograph can also serve as proof that your stalker tried to approach you.

- Consider buying or renting a video surveillance camera. Install it inside or outside your home. If your stalker approaches you, vandalizes your property, or simply leaves you a letter or gift, you may be able to capture it on tape.

4. Contact the police. Don't wait until the stalking turns threatening or violent to contact law enforcement. Even if the police do not take immediate action, you will be establishing an official police record of the stalking.

Bring a typewritten description of the stalking with you which you have prepared ahead of time. A police station can be a very stressful environment, and with only your memory to rely upon, you may forget important details; also, you may be too emotional to relate your story clearly. A written timeline and description gets around both problems: it transcends emotion and gives police the facts they really need.

5. Contact a lawyer. Hire one privately, or explore the low-cost or no-cost services of Legal Aid. If possible, find an attorney who is sympathetic to your situation, and understands the stalking laws in your state. Have him or her send a "cease and desist" letter to your stalker (via registered mail, so you'll have proof that he received it). This puts your stalker on notice that you're prepared to enlist outside support.

If your stalker is arrested, don't assume that you no longer need an attorney. You may have to take an active role in the legal process in order to protect yourself. For example, because many stalking behaviors are charged as misdemeanors, your stalker may be released "on his own recognizance" unless you and your attorney argue against it.

Don't wait until the stalking escalates before contacting a lawyer.

At the first sign of stalking behavior, make a strong, preemptive strike. There are no guarantees that a cease and desist letter will solve your problem; third-party intervention provokes as many stalkers as it deters. Yet it can sometimes nip the stalking in the bud. At the very least, it lays a foundation of written evidence, evidence that will strengthen your case if you pursue further legal action.

6. "Tell the world." A woman is often too embarrassed or ashamed to tell other people that she is being stalked. (This is especially true if the stalker is the woman's former husband or boyfriend.) Guilt is another common reaction; the victim blames the stalking on something *she* said or did. So she says nothing to anyone. She keeps the problem to herself.

The stalker counts on this reaction. If you're ever stalked, therefore, do not keep it private. Do the unexpected: tell the world. "Publicize" every instance of stalking behavior, and every encounter you have with the stalker. Tell anyone and everyone. Bring your problem out into the open.

Ask others to inform you if your stalker turns up where you live or work. Give them his description and (ideally) his photograph. Don't be afraid to request specific kinds of assistance: for example, you might ask a co-worker to walk you to your car each night, or ask a neighbor to keep an eye on your home and property. Finally, make it clear to others that they should not give out any personal information about you: where you live or work, who your friends are, and so on.

While some people may react to your claims with skepticism, the law of averages dictates that the more people you tell, the more likely you are to find people who *will* give you practical assistance and vital emotional support. So whatever you do, don't try to carry the whole burden alone. Enlisting the help of others is not a sign of weakness, but a sign of strength. It's a way of taking action and exercising your own power.

7. Get a restraining order. This should cover all types of stalking behavior: not just following you or approaching you, but calling you by phone, trespassing on your property, and sending or delivering you mail or gifts. Depending on the state you live in and the specific conditions of the restraining order, it may also be called a "no-contact," "stay away" or "anti-stalking" order, or an "order of protection."

Some experts believe that a restraining order is just as likely to provoke a stalker as deter him. Indeed, some stalkers do perceive restraining orders as a challenge and resort to violence to demonstrate their defiance, so you should take this into consideration when deciding whether or not to get one. At the same time, however, keep in mind that a restraining order does have several recognizable benefits. It becomes part of an official police record on the stalker. It empowers police to make an arrest if the order is violated. It can empower the district attorney to charge further instances of stalking as felonies, rather than as misdemeanors. Finally, a restraining order can be invaluable in cases where it's your word against his. Many stalkers talk their way out of arrest by convincing police that he and the victim are just having a "lover's spat," or by portraying the victim as paranoid or hysterical. Presenting a restraining order will make it crystal-clear to police that this is not the case.

8. Get professional help. Stalking takes a tremendous emotional toll on its victim. In addition to enlisting help from your friends and loved ones, therefore, try to join a support group or get professional therapy. Do this in any case, but especially if you are showing symptoms of rage, depression, or stress.

9. Use your anger. If you are targeted by a stalker, anger is one emotion you are almost guaranteed to feel. This anger can be either a blessing or a curse, depending on how you channel it.

- DON'T let your anger "explode" towards everyone around you: unsympathetic friends or relatives, for example, or police who refuse to take action. Instead, channel it into appropriate action, and direct it solely towards your stalker.
- DON'T act rashly by trying to take the law into your own hands. Don't try to turn the tables by following, harassing, or threatening your stalker; you may escalate the situation and put yourself at greater risk.

- DON'T let anger make you so cocky, defiant, or full of bravado ("I'll show *him!*") that you lose your objectivity. Any stalking situation is potentially dangerous; it's impossible to predict what may put another person over the edge.
- DON'T turn your anger inward and blame yourself for the problem.

10. Protect yourself. Exercise an extra degree of caution to protect yourselves and your loved ones.

The Illusion of Empowerment: Examining Guns, Sprays, and Other Weapons

It never fails: every time I speak on the subject of personal empowerment, someone in the audience will ask, "Should I carry a weapon?" And my answer to that question usually runs along the lines of "Yes, you should . . . and no, you shouldn't."

Don't get me wrong. I'm not completely opposed to guns or to protective devices like pepper spray; in certain situations, "external" weapons can be of real value. What I do oppose is the idea that any external weapon can take the place of empowerment that comes from within. I'm convinced that while a weapon can sometimes be used as an extension of your personal power, *it can never be a substitute for it.*

In the past 10 years, we've seen a boom in the market for firearms and protective devices. Yet I believe that the most valuable weapons in your arsenal can't be bought at a gun store or through a mail-order catalogue. I'm referring to "power tools" like intuition, verbal skills like de-escalation and verbal self-defense, and your own natural weapons like hands, feet, and teeth, just to name a few. These are your true first lines of defense, yet most people don't even know that they have them (much less know how to use them). Lacking this knowledge, they look to external devices to ensure their safety.

Unfortunately, any device has certain limitations. Unlike your natural weapons, a gun, stun gun, or canister of chemical spray can be taken away from you, and possibly used against you. It can malfunction or misfire. You can forget to carry it, or be unable to get to it in a crisis. When a weapon is your only line of defense, it's all too easy to become defenseless.

Relying on a weapon is also like relying on another person to protect you: whether it's a stun gun or a big, strong man, they're both crutches. And like all crutches, they can serve to impair your personal empowerment rather than enhance it. With the false sense of security that a weapon can bestow, you're less likely to develop and use all your other options.

Buying a protective device can seem like a quick fix, an instant, easy answer to the problem of personal protection. Indeed, most advertising for protective devices emphasizes how inexpensive they are to buy and how simple they are to use. Another "advantage" you often see promoted is the fact that a woman can use a protective device without having to get close to her attacker. She sees him approaching, she raises her arm, and—WHAM!—debilitates him with a dose of pepper spray. Point and shoot; impersonal self-defense at its finest. Unfortunately, this isn't realistic in most cases. What if you don't see your attacker coming? You have neither the time nor the opportunity to discharge your weapon. And because you've relied on your weapon to protect you, you have nothing else to fall back on.

When I was 5 years old, I came very close to drowning. My family was vacationing on a lake. I hadn't yet learned to swim, but I boldly decided one morning to put an inner tube around my waist and venture out above my head. Little did I know, the inner tube had a leak; it began to noticeably deflate when I was fairly far from shore. It was only through sheer luck that my father was outside looking for me and happened to hear my shouts for help. A minute more and I would have been in serious trouble.

In recent years, I've come to see my "near death experience" as something of a metaphor for the way we can put too much reliance on external means of protection. As a child, I placed all my reliance on a device; when it failed, I had no inner resources (namely, the ability to swim!) to fall back on. As an adult, I'm determined to never repeat that same mistake.

So as I describe the pros and cons of various weapons, never forget one thing: a weapon is a device, nothing more, nothing less. It should never take the place of your mind, heart, intuition, and natural weapons.

Guns

A few years back, I ran into a woman I'd known from college. When our conversation turned towards my line of work, Natalie evinced polite interest in the subject of "personal empowerment for women," but insisted that she would never be interested in learning the techniques of physical self-defense. She was so insistent, in fact, that I finally had to ask, "Well, why not?" She smiled and said, "Because I don't need to. You see, *I own a gun.*"

Natalie isn't the first person I've met who believes in the invincibility of guns, and I doubt that she'll be the last. Guns are associated with power. And although the NRA insists that "Guns don't kill people, people kill people," the fact remains that guns are extremely lethal. They're easy to conceal, easy to carry, and take little or no physical strength to fire. They can be fired from a distance, yet inflict devastating injuries.

However, gun ownership carries its own particular risks. Statistics show that a gun purchased for home protection is more likely to kill a family member than an intruder. If a woman has a live-in partner, for example, and they have a gun in the house, her partner is more likely to use the gun against *her* than against an intruder (especially if he has a history of domestic abuse). And each year, hundreds of children are accidentally killed by guns that their parents believed to be unloaded, locked away, or safely out of reach.

I have no objection to buying a gun for home protection if you live alone (no children, no live-in partner), have no mental illness (including clinical depression), and are well-trained in the use of firearms. Even in those circumstances, I believe that your gun has to be loaded, ready, and within reach to make a real difference. Think about it: if you wake to find an intruder in your bedroom, chances are you won't have the opportunity to get to any gun that is locked in a cabinet, stored in a closet, or even kept in a bedside drawer. And even in situations where you have a few seconds warning—if your security system goes off, for example, or you hear an intruder downstairs—I'd rather see you get to a designated "safe room" and call the police than confront the intruder yourself.

I don't believe that anyone, man or woman, should carry a gun in public, not even in his or her car. (The one possible exception: if a woman is being stalked, and believes her life to be in danger.) Although it is legal to carry a licensed firearm in some states, I believe that the person who does so is less likely to use their other resources, such as awareness and intuition, and less likely to try other methods to resolve conflicts.

Some survivors of violent crime purchase a gun to help them feel less vulnerable, less helpless, and more in control. Although I understand their motives, no weapon should take the place of professional counseling and therapy. Rather than helping the healing process, possession of a gun may hinder it because the gun conveys the illusion of empowerment.

If you are seriously considering purchasing a handgun, I urge you to learn more about the subject. Of all the books that discuss gun ownership for women, Paxton Quigley's *Armed and Female* is probably the most thorough. Although I don't share her enthusiasm for firearms, Quigley does provide essential information about buying a gun and learning how to use it. She also discusses the legal and moral responsibilities that come with owning a firearm.

Nonlethal Weapons

Pepper spray. For many years, mace was the most common type of chemical self-defense spray. In recent years, however, it has been overtaken in popularity by pepper spray, and for good reason. Unlike mace (which is essentially a form of tear gas), pepper spray can instantly incapacitate your attacker. In addition to acute eye irritation, it can cause gagging, uncontrollable coughing, breathing difficulties, and intense pain.

Pepper spray can be very effective, but only if you use it properly. If you carry it in public, it must be in your hand, armed and ready; if you carry it in your pocket or your purse, you probably won't get to it in time. You must spray it in your attacker's *face,* ideally from around five feet away; if you're too far from your attacker, or so close that the ingredients are unable to mix properly, pepper spray may be ineffective. You must remember to aim it in the right direction; in the heat of the moment, many people have forgotten this and sprayed *themselves* instead. If you use it indoors, or outdoors when the wind is blowing in your direction, you may suffer some or even most of its effects. And like any other weapon, the canister may be knocked out of your hand; some statistics show that this happens in fully *half* of situations where pepper spray is involved. Your attacker may also get a hold of it and turn it against you.

If you decide to carry pepper spray, get some hands-on training in how to use it; manufacturers' simplistic "point and shoot" directions are often inadequate.

Stun Guns. Stun guns are not guns in the conventional sense of the word, but rather small, battery-powered devices that produce an electronic discharge. At 65,000 volts, a stun gun will cause painful muscle spasms; at 200,000 volts, it can incapacitate a person for up to 10 minutes. You have to get close to use a stun gun, and you should always bring it up your attacker's blind side. Stun guns are scary-looking (when activated, a visible charge of electricity travels across the electrodes) so they have some deterrent value as well.

The limitations of a stun gun? You can forget to carry it. It can malfunction. It may be knocked from your hand. It may be used against you. You have to press it hard against your attacker's body for several seconds, which can seem like an eternity in an assault situation. Finally, stun guns don't incapacitate everyone they're used against; no two people react the same to them (so if you're going to buy one, buy the one with the most voltage).

Taser Guns. Sold as a nonlethal weapon, taser guns use either gun powder (law enforcement-issued only) or compressed air to launch two electrical probes attached to a wire of up to 15 feet long. The probes will stick to skin or clothing, allowing the user to incapacitate an attacker from a distance by delivering an electrical current with effects similar to that of a stun gun.

In recent years the taser gun has grown in popularity, but has come under fire by some in the law enforcement community. In addition to concerns that this weapon may fall into the hands of criminals, some worry that the taser gun may prove lethal if used against children, the elderly, or someone with heart or other health-related problems.

Like other external weapons, the taser gun can malfunction or be used against you. It's also expensive, costing anywhere from $200 to $400. Banned in some states, it's advised that you check with your local police department for the laws pertaining to the purchase and use of this weapon.

Kubotans. The kubotan is *my* external weapon of choice; I carry it on my key ring, so I always have it with me when I'm out in public. Despite its exotic-sounding name, a kubotan is a very simple object: a mini-baton approximately three-and-a-half inches long, with a ribbed surface and a hole through one end so you can attach it to your key ring. Designed by a martial arts instructor, kubotans are carried by law enforcement professionals, such as prison guards and police. Inexpensive to buy ($2 to $5) and easy to carry, they come in plastic, wood, or metal. (A word of caution: a metal kubotan may be confiscated by airport security.)

If you carry a kubotan in public, carry it in your hand. You want it at your fingertips, not buried in your jacket pocket or purse. To use it properly, you need to get close to your attacker, but that's fine, too: you've already learned the advantages of getting close. Bring it up your attacker's blind side and jab it into his eye, throat, ribs, bladder, groin, or thigh. Like a pen or a pencil, it can be used for both attention-getter and vital-target attacks. Keep it on your key ring at all times.

A word about keys themselves. Because most of us carry a set of keys when we're out in public, women are often advised to use them as weapons (placing one key between their fingers with the sharp end pointed out). However, this is very poor self-defense advice. It's very difficult to grip a key this way, and you're just as likely to scrape your own hand in the process. My recommendation is to attach some other kind of weapon to your key ring, preferably a kubotan.

Note: Pepper spray canisters are widely available; they can be purchased by mail order, at gun stores, and at many hardware stores and sporting goods outlets. Stun guns are sold at gun stores and some electronics stores; taser guns are sold at selected electronics and sporting good stores; kubatons can be purchased at gun stores and martial arts supply stores.

To the Rescue: Interceding in Assault Situations

Throughout this book, I've emphasized over and over that your primary goal during any assault is to get to safety as soon as possible. But how does this apply if you witness an assault upon someone else? How do you reconcile the need to protect yourself with the admirable desire to help another person?

No matter who you are, from elderly woman to off-duty police officer, any intervention can be risky. However, there are ways to intercede without taking needless risks. If you follow some basic guidelines, in other words, you can help another person without becoming a victim yourself.

In my opinion, the single most important thing to consider when it comes to intervention is the ever-present possibility that the attacker has a weapon. If the attacker is armed—and *especially* if he has a gun—you might be injured or killed just for verbally intervening, or even for daring to get too close. (Believe me, it happens all too often.) So unless you are absolutely sure that the attacker is unarmed, *keep a safe distance* and employ other methods to deter the assault.

Use distraction. The idea is to do anything that may divert the attacker's attention away from his victim. So make noise: honk your car horn, set off your car alarm, and use your voice (call, yell, rant, rave: it's all distraction). And don't stop there. Throw a rock through a business's plate-glass window; the sound of breaking glass is itself distracting and might also set off the store's alarm system. If it's after dark, train your headlights on the attacker, and flick them off and on. In addition to distracting him, these kinds of techniques may also attract the attention of other people.

Remain on the scene. Many witnesses to assault leave the scene to call the police, believing that this is the very best way to help the victim. Unfortunately, by the time they find a pay phone and make the call, and by the time the police arrive, the assault is usually over. The victim has already been injured, abducted, or killed, and there's not much left to do but call an ambulance. And because witnesses often leave the crime scene prematurely, they're unable to supply police with much useful information, such as a license plate number, or a description of the attacker.

Whenever possible, therefore, persuade another person to leave and call police while you yourself remain at the crime scene. (Unless you have a cellular phone, which would allow you to do *both*.) Even if you're the only witness, you should still remain on the scene. If the attacker tries to move his victim, move with him. If he forces her into a car, get in your own car and stay on his tail. Don't underestimate the deterrent value your very presence may have on the attacker.

Don't assume that somebody else will intervene. Even if other people are around, they may do *nothing* at all to help; a sad reality, but a reality nonetheless. You might recall the notorious case in 1964 of Kitty Genovese, chased, stabbed, chased again, and finally killed while 38 neighbors heard but ignored her terrified screams for help. Genovese's experience has become far too typical. In one recent case in Oakland, California, a woman was raped, taken at knifepoint into a liquor store, and then beaten, while two clerks watched but did nothing. As this woman said, *"I never expected them to risk their lives. I just wanted them to call 911 and hit the panic button under the register."*

There are many reasons why witnesses may do nothing. They may not care enough to get involved, be too scared to intervene, or be too paralyzed by shock to do anything at all. Their willingness to intercede may also depend on the relative "weakness" of the victim; for example, people are more likely to intercede to help a child than to help an adult, and (rightly or wrongly) may be more apt to help a woman than a man.

People may also be reluctant to intervene if the attacker and victim appear to know one another. If a man hits his wife or girlfriend in public, for example, witnesses may perceive the assault as being "only" a family argument or lovers' quarrel. Even if they do try to intercede, the attacker (and sometimes the victim) may tell them to mind their own business, as if the assault is a "private matter" and not really a criminal act.

Because of all these factors, you should be prepared for two distinct possibilities in any intervention situation: one, if you don't intercede, there's a good chance that no one else will; two, if you do intercede, you may very well be doing it alone.

If you witness an assault and you're convinced that the attacker *doesn't* have a weapon, you have some additional options. You can remain on the scene, use distraction, and leave it at that, but you can also get close and take a more assertive approach. You can try verbal techniques such as de-escalation or verbal self-defense; after all, getting involved doesn't necessarily mean getting physical. At the same time, however, I wouldn't rule out some form of physical intervention if you feel it will make a difference.

As you've learned by now, it doesn't matter how big or strong he is: any unarmed attacker is vulnerable to effective counterattack. And whether you're intervening on another person's behalf, or fighting to defend yourself, the principles of self-defense remain the same. So if you do choose to physically intervene, forget about fighting against the attacker's strength by trying to pull him off, or drag him away from his victim. Instead, cause pain. Think back to the attention-getters and vital-target attacks that you have learned.

One decided advantage you might have is the ability to surprise the attacker from behind. You can kick him in the calf, or in the back of the knee. In a more serious situation, you can reach around his head and dig your fingers into his eyes. One behind-the-back technique that works particularly well is to comb your hands through his hair, grab hold, then forcefully pull back and *down* along his spine. This is the easiest way to separate an attacker from his intended victim. You'll be controlling his head, and where the head goes, the body follows. This technique works whether the attacker is on his feet or on the ground (as in a rape attempt). And believe me, it will cause pain!

In the end, choosing to intercede or not is a moral decision that is yours alone to make. Altruism has to be weighed against self-preservation, apathy against heroism; however you choose to look at it, it presents some tricky moral dilemmas that I would encourage you to examine *now,* before an assault takes place. Assaults can occur at lightning speed; split-second decisions must be made, and action quickly taken. That's why I believe it's important to think ahead, to ask yourself, "Under what circumstances would I risk my personal safety? Just how far would I go to help another person?"

Imagine, for example, that you're in a park one sunny day when someone tries to abduct or abuse your child. Would you try to physically intervene? Absolutely! And you'd probably do the same thing even if the child were not your own. But what if the victim was a woman, or a man? And what if the attacker had a knife, or had a gun? What if the attack occurred late at night, or in a bad neighborhood? And what if you weren't alone, but had your children with you? Would their presence make you any less willing to intercede?

These are just some of the many factors to consider when deciding to intervene. Think about them now; waiting until an actual crisis occurs may be waiting too late.

13
TAKING THE NEXT STEP

Getting An Early Start: Empowering Our Daughters

It's never too late to learn about personal empowerment and self-defense. I've taught women in their 70s and 80s and seen them acquire the same level of confidence, assertiveness, and physical skills as students half their age. But if it's never too late to learn, it's also never too early to start. Time and again, my students have said they wished they'd acquired this knowledge sooner. As one woman told me, "If I'd learned this stuff as a teenager, it would have changed the rest of my life."

Unfortunately, the idea of teaching young girls how to protect themselves effectively continues to be devalued. Some people actually disapprove of it, believing that the young girl trained in self-defense will be more likely to get herself into situations "over her head," or that the girl who can fight is somehow less feminine. The attitude of many parents is that while boys should learn to protect themselves, girls should be protected. Or to put it another way, that boys should learn to be self-reliant, but girls should learn to be cautious. Unfortunately, those same girls must eventually leave home. And when they do, they leave with little to protect them but a warning to "be careful."

I believe that *all* children and adolescents should be given some basic, age-appropriate instruction in how to defend themselves. A girl is never too young to become an active participant in her own protection. Start early, and you set her on the road towards becoming a woman who will not only be adept at defending herself verbally and physically, but confident in her ability to do so.

The value of teaching your daughter self-defense doesn't begin and end with protecting her from violent crime: from the rapist, kidnapper, or child molester. She will also be able to defend herself from a schoolyard bully or an abusive boyfriend. Among my female students, most can recall being harassed, bullied, or even physically assaulted (shoved, tripped, etc.) during childhood, and how weak and helpless they were made to feel. Experiences like these have a lasting impact; feelings of powerlessness can persist into adulthood and contribute to a woman's poor self-image. As they learn about empowerment and self-defense, my students invariably look back to their childhoods and say, "If I'd only known then what I know now." They realize they could have handled many incidents differently, or avoided them altogether. All they lacked at the time was *knowledge*.

We can't change the past, but we can help the next generation. No one should have to tolerate mistreatment, and teaching a daughter about empowerment and self-defense is one of the most loving things a parent can do. Here are some ideas on how to get her started.

1. Teach by example. Your daughter learns a lot by watching how you interact with other people. Are you passive by nature? Cautious, fearful, averse to confrontation? Do you ask for male help to handle "ugly" situations? Do you get overly upset when a stranger is nasty or rude to you? If the answer to any of these questions is "yes," you may be sending the wrong message.

Maybe you tend instead towards the other extreme. Unfortunately, this has its own disadvantages. For example, Judy's mother was a forceful, strong-minded woman, the proverbial tigress ready to defend her young, and Judy could still remember watching as her mother gave tongue-lashings to shop clerks, schoolteachers, or virtually anyone who crossed her. Yet instead of being impressed or inspired by these displays, Judy was mortified by them. She cringed in embarrassment. Today, Judy is a quiet, timid, soft-spoken woman, who by her own admission dreads confrontation and is far too eager to please. And she feels that one reason she became that way was because she didn't want to be like her mother. Her childhood experiences had led her to believe that the only way to be assertive was to be aggressive, that assertiveness was a harsh and unattractive quality.

The best way for a girl to learn to be self-reliant and assertive is from her parents' example, and particularly from her mother's. Nothing takes the place of a positive role model.

2. Encourage physical activities. Girls should be encouraged to participate in sports as much as boys are, and that doesn't mean they have to take up boxing or football. There are plenty of team sports (basketball, baseball, soccer) and individual ones (tennis, swimming, gymnastics) that serve the same purpose: developing a girl's natural physical abilities and the self-confidence and self-esteem that go with it.

3. Teach your daughter how to communicate. Preschool teachers know the importance of verbal skills; that's why they teach students to "use their words" instead of pushing, kicking, or biting to get their way. If only more adults followed that advice! Clear communication is essential in resolving and avoiding conflict. Children who are poor at communicating verbally are more likely to get into fights.

Once children start attending school, their first encounter with physical aggression usually comes in the form of the playground bully. You can help your child deal with a bully by teaching her how to communicate. Give her specific words and phrases to use; "Stop bothering me," "Go away," and "Back off," are all fine examples. For younger children, the "Stop it or . . ." response works well, as in "Stop it or I won't play with you," or "Stop it or I'm going home."

And teach your daughter that whatever her choice of words, her message must be delivered firmly and *calmly* to be effective: displays of emotion only reward the bully and therefore make things worse. Teach her how to feign indifference, to shrug or laugh off minor taunts. And emphasize that it's okay to walk away from some bullies or avoid them altogether; she doesn't have to "win" every confrontation.

At the same time, let your daughter know that the value of strong verbal skills extends well beyond confrontational situations. Encourage her to be assertive in all her interactions with others; teach her that she can speak up and be direct. Even today, girls are often encouraged to use charm, flattery, "feminine wiles," and other indirect means to get what they want; unfortunately, this implies that they will be ineffective—and perceived as unfeminine—if they take a more direct and assertive approach.

Along these lines, I recall something told me by a friend who'd been raised in the Deep South. Almost from birth, Lydia had been conditioned to believe that because she was a girl, subtle forms of manipulation were the key to getting what she wanted and she carried that conditioning into adulthood. "Al," she said, "let me tell you how I was taught to communicate. If I was driving down the road with my husband and I started to get thirsty, I wouldn't say 'I'm getting thirsty.' I'd smile and say, 'Honey, you're looking a little parched. Why don't we stop so's I can get you a nice cold drink?' "

There's nothing wrong with diplomacy, and most of us use it all the time. Yet it's important to communicate to girls that being direct is one of their prerogatives, and frankness and positive assertiveness can often be the better way to go.

4. Teach your daughter verbal self-defense. As children, most of us can recall being told never to talk to strangers. While that principle still makes sense—avoiding unnecessary dialogue with strangers *is* a good idea—it does need to be expanded. As victims of incest and child molestation have taught us, a child is just as likely to be threatened by someone he or she knows as by a stranger. Meanwhile, children who are taught to keep quiet and never challenge an adult's authority run a greater risk of being molested or abducted, as do children who are reticent and shy.

So a better maxim for our children is this: if anyone speaks to them, touches them, or approaches them in an inappropriate way, they should verbally protest loudly and vigorously! Role-playing exercises are a particularly effective way of getting this lesson across. With you playing the role of the aggressor, encourage your child to look you in the eye and issue commands that are short and direct: "Let me go!", "Go away!", "Back off!", and so on. And have her practice yelling "No!" at the top of her voice.

If a stranger tries to abduct your child, your child should make it clear to anyone who may be within earshot that the abductor is not a parent, friend, or baby-sitter. Without this clarification, other people may feel uncertain about intervening; after all, how many times have you seen a parent carry a toddler out of a store as the child screams "No, no, no!" Therefore, teach your child to say things like, "Let me go! I don't know you!" and "Go away! You're not my mommy/daddy!"

There is one way in which verbal self-defense for children differs from that for teenagers or adults: I wouldn't advise any child to *step forward* as he or she delivers a statement or "command." In the case of children, "moving in the right direction" means running from an aggressor at the first available opportunity.

5. Teach your daughter how to fight. In a perfect world, neither boys nor girls would need to know how to fight, and I am the last person to encourage aggressiveness of any kind. But the fact remains that children *can* find themselves physically threatened. This may run the gamut from a slap from a schoolyard bully, to abduction or molestation at the hands of an adult. Unfortunately, while most boys get some experience fighting or wrestling as kids, girls are usually discouraged from ever attempting it. Instead, we encourage them to play it safe. As a result, many girls grow up believing that they are physically incapable of protecting themselves.

The last decade has seen an explosion in karate classes for small children. The idea makes some people uncomfortable, as though the goal of these classes is to turn out pint-sized Ninjas who will terrorize other children. In reality, however, these classes are valuable for the restraint, discipline, and respect for others that they instill in their students.

Denise, the 6-year-old daughter of a friend of mine, asked to take karate classes after seeing her older brother do so. Though initially skeptical, her parents finally gave their permission, in part because Denise had recently become the target of a bully at school.

(Yes, it starts that early.) A month into her training, Denise was physically threatened by that same bully. Did she retaliate with a swift kick or karate chop? Quite the opposite: she looked him in the eye and said firmly but calmly, "Go away. I'm not afraid of you." *And it worked.* Why? Because Denise wasn't bluffing; she really wasn't afraid. She knew she had the physical skills to back up her words.

A good martial arts program teaches children how to use their words, and how to walk away from provocation. They learn to employ physical retaliation only as the very last resort. They're less likely to get into fights, and less likely to be victimized. So if you're planning to send your daughter to ballet classes and your son to karate, you might want to rethink your decision. In my opinion, your daughter needs that self-defense training just as much as your son does.

6. Teach your daughter *when* to fight. In 1995, after hearing me lecture to a group of educators, one high school teacher approached me to report the following: in recent years, she and her colleagues had seen a dramatic rise in incidents of teenage girls kicking male schoolmates in the groin. Many of these attacks had resulted in serious physical injury.

Was this good news? Did it signify a healthy trend away from "victimhood" and towards personal empowerment? Absolutely not! If anything, it was a horrifying example of "assertiveness" and "feminism" being grossly misinterpreted. Because in almost every case, those attacks were initiated in response to purely *verbal* provocation (threats, harassment, etc.). Those girls weren't using self-defense, but misusing it.

Hand in hand with learning any physical technique is knowing when and when not to use it. Alas, while some of the things we teach our children are etched in black and white (*"Never* play with matches"), teaching a daughter how to respond to provocation, threats, or physical aggression will never be so simple; every situation she encounters will be unique, and must be judged accordingly. By way of illustration, I'd like you to imagine the following scenario:

Twelve-year-old Karen is walking home from school. As she passes by a group of male classmates, one sticks out his foot and trips her to the ground. The other boys burst out laughing.

What should Karen do? Breaking into tears or running off won't solve anything, so that leaves her with three remaining options. She could get to her feet and calmly keep on walking. She could retaliate physically with a well-placed attention-getter, or even a knee to the groin. Or she could walk back to the boy, look him straight in the eye, and make a calm but definitive statement (not a threat), e.g. "I won't allow you to hurt me," or simply "Don't ever do that again."

Each response has its pros and cons, and each might have different repercussions. For example, if Karen were to keep on walking, the boy might interpret her exit as a sign of weakness (result: he trips her again the next day); on the other hand, it might just as easily deprive him of any satisfaction (result: he's discouraged from trying it again). Physical retaliation might get Karen into hot water with the principal, make her a target of schoolyard teasing ("Ooooh, here comes big bad Karen . . ."), or even cause the boy's friends to join into the fight; however, the boy might also get the message that Karen will never allow him to hurt her (result: he never does it again). Verbal confrontation might escalate the situation (result: the boy shoves Karen to the ground); on the other hand, it might convince him that Karen is not a good target (result: no further harassment).

In my opinion, verbal confrontation *would* be Karen's best option in this particular situation. She wouldn't be backing down, but taking assertive action. She'd be delivering a warning ("Don't ever do that again") without delivering a provocative threat or ultimatum (". . . or you'll be sorry").

But whatever my opinion or yours, here's the bottom line: only Karen can decide which is the right response for her. No one can tell her ahead of time what to do or not to do in every single situation; there are just too many variables. For example, if that boy had tripped Karen as a prelude to further assault, a physical response might have been not just appropriate, but essential. If he'd simply jostled her, however, and she wasn't really hurt, verbal confrontation might have been more in order. Remember, self-defense is designed to protect you from physical harm, not from every push, shove or nudge you might encounter. (And that's as true for adults as it is for children!) On the other hand, if Karen had been tripped while in a bad neighborhood, or by a boy she didn't recognize, her intuition might have told her to avoid any interaction, to leave the scene and get to safety as quickly as possible.

As Karen's story illustrates, there are no one-size-fits-all solutions when it comes to personal empowerment. Therefore, the most important way you can empower your daughter is by giving her the tools she will need to make the right decisions. Share with her the many lessons provided throughout this book. Teach her the value of objectivity, and encourage her to trust her own intuition. And remember: decision-making is a skill that no one masters overnight, so start this process now. Someday your daughter will thank you for it.

Personal Empowerment for Teenagers

The American Association of University Women has identified some types of sexually-related harassment that teenage girls encounter. These include:

- Sexual comments, jokes, gestures or looks
- Sexual pictures, notes, and graffiti
- Sexual rumors about them (that they are lesbian, frigid, promiscuous, etc.)
- Flashing or mooning
- Being touched, grabbed, or pinched in a sexual way
- Having their clothing pulled down or off
- Being blocked or cornered by a sexually aggressive date
- Being forced to kiss a boy or perform some other sexual act

Pretty horrifying, isn't it? When I show that same list to my female students, they all remember having endured at least one of those forms of harassment. And many of them are mothers who'd do just about anything to break the cycle and protect their daughters from similar treatment.

Fortunately, the teenage girl today has some options that didn't exist for her mother. For many years, society's attitude towards harassment of teenage girls was that "boys will be boys," and enduring their "pranks" a regrettable yet unavoidable part of adolescence. Recently, however, some schools have started to take the issue more seriously. I support this trend wholeheartedly: harassment is as much a disciplinary problem as fighting in the schoolyard or destroying school property, and there's no reason to tolerate it. A harasser is a harasser whether he's 17 or 37, and whether the harassment takes place in the schoolyard or the workplace.

Once again, however, we run the risk of depending on higher authorities to solve all our problems. Our ultimate goal should not be to protect our daughters, but to teach them how to protect themselves. Earlier in this book, I urged you to try handling confrontations yourself before "running for help": to confront a sexual harasser on the job, for example, before filing a sexual harassment suit. If your teenage daughter is being harassed or bullied, the same rule applies: *she* should take the first steps towards stopping it. She will discover that doing so can be an empowering experience, and in most cases, will stop the harassment right in its tracks. If the harassment does continue (and especially if it escalates), she can still ask you or school authorities to intervene. Let her know she always has "backup" if she needs it.

I'm not saying parents should throw caution to the wind and abdicate their roles as protectors. But there's a real difference between protection and overprotection; one is supportive, the other debilitating. And when girls reach puberty, we tend to overprotect them. We encourage them to run for help instead of fostering self-reliance. As columnist Chiori Santiago writes, "As teenagers, boys earn more freedom and privileges, girls become more cloistered. Boys are taught to face the world with courage; girls are taught to view it with fear." That may protect girls in the short-term, but it doesn't prepare them for real life.

There was a time when I congratulated myself on my protective attitude towards women. If a woman asked for my help in dealing with a harasser, for example, I was always quick to say, "I'll handle him for you." In retrospect, I realize how patronizing that attitude really was. Yet with the best of intentions, parents often fall into the same trap.

Today, if I had a girlfriend who was being harassed, I'd encourage her to first try handling the situation on her own. And I encourage all of you parents to instill that same self-reliance in your daughters. That will help them far more in the long run than any short-term intervention you might offer. Yes, girls are more at risk for certain types of assault, and the fear that our daughters will be sexually assaulted has a basis in reality. But school is a microcosm of the outside world, and the teenage years a training ground for adulthood. If you want your daughter to grow to be an assertive, capable, and independent woman, start encouraging her in that direction now.

The Safety Factor: Your Personal Daily Checklist

The following checklist provides some specific safety and security measures to take in your home and workplace, in your car and on the street, and while traveling out of town. Many of these measures are based on simple common sense; others draw on the expertise of law enforcement and home security professionals. **Note:** For a more comprehensive look at crime prevention, I highly recommend Ira A. Lipman's *How to Protect Yourself From Crime.*

Above any empowerment techniques, preventive measures still remain your best defense. At the same time, remember that your intuition is still the single most effective "safety device" that you have in your possession.

SAFETY AT HOME

Make your home secure:

- Consider installing a security system. It should cover *all* entry points into your home, including windows.
- If possible, buy a dog. A barking dog is a deterrent to many

intruders, and even a small dog can serve as an excellent "early warning system."

- Consider having your local police department or a private security service provide a safety evaluation of your home.
- Install deadbolts on all exterior doors. Keep exterior doors and windows locked at all times.
- Keep the exterior of your home well-lit. Darkness favors the home intruder.
- Keep the entrance to your home free of any obstructions, such as heavy shrubbery. Some home intruders lie in wait, then, when the homeowner returns home and unlocks the door, they force their way inside.
- Consider the advantage of portable phones. A portable phone can be carried outside the house, or from room to room, in the event of an emergency.
- If you can afford to buy one, keep a working cellular phone in your home. Be aware that conventional phone lines can go down, or be deliberately cut.

Exercise caution at home:

- Never let anyone know that you are home alone.
- Never open your door to a stranger. Install a peephole. Remember that some secondary doors (e.g. screen doors or glass storm doors) can give an illusion of safety without truly protecting you: glass can be shattered, and the flimsy mesh of some screen doors can be punched through or ripped away.
- Never allow a repairperson, meter reader, or utility company employee into your home unless you've made prior arrangements with his or her office. Always ask to see photo identification. While any stranger is inside your home, be aware of where he or she is at all times.
- Always use an initial rather than a first name for building directories, mailboxes, and telephone listings.
- Take note of any unusual activity in your neighborhood: moving vans, outside workers, delivery persons or vehicles.
- Participate in a neighborhood watch group.

Phone safety:

- Consider having an unlisted number.
- Instruct everyone you live with (husband, children, roommate) not to give out personal information over the phone. Never participate in phone surveys, or confirm your phone number to a caller who has called you "by mistake."
- Whether you live alone or not, your outgoing answering machine message should always begin with "We're not available . . ." rather than "I'm not at home . . ."

If you leave the house:

- Keep a light and radio turned on while you're away.
- When you return home, always have your housekey or apartment key in hand.
- If you return home and spot something unusual—front door ajar, window broken or open—DO NOT ENTER TO INVESTIGATE. Get to a safe place, then call the police.
- If you go away on vacation, stop delivery of your newspapers, and arrange for someone to pick up your mail each day. Install automatic switches (time-activated or light-sensitive) to illuminate your house after dark.

Prepare for home emergencies:

- Teach your children how to dial 911. Make sure they know their address and telephone number.
- Have a detailed escape plan. Whether the threat comes from a fire or a home intruder, everyone in the family should know how to get out of the house. They should also know where to go or regroup once they have gotten outside.

  Currently on the market are some safety ladders which can be unrolled out of an upstairs window. These ladders, however, can be extremely difficult to negotiate, especially if you're elderly or have a child in your arms. A better idea is to have a strong, thick rope, knotted at regular intervals. It's actually much easier to lower yourself down a knotted rope than to climb down a ladder.

If you see or hear an intruder in your home:

- DO NOT GO TO INVESTIGATE. Get out of the house and go elsewhere to call for assistance.
- If you look outside and see someone trying to steal your car, DO NOT GO OUTSIDE. Many car thieves are armed, so stay inside and call the police.
- Designate one room on each floor as a "safe room" for situations where you cannot safely leave your home: if you are upstairs, for example, when you hear an intruder downstairs. This room ideally should have a strong door, a deadbolt, a working flashlight, and cellular phone. In the event of an intruder or a domestic abuse emergency, retreat to this room and call the police.

SAFETY IN PUBLIC

While on foot:

- Stay alert and conscious of your surroundings at all times.
- Remember that there's always more safety in numbers. Avoid walking alone whenever possible. If you exercise outdoors, do it with a friend.
- Wear flat shoes or sneakers whenever possible.
- Use well-traveled and well-lit streets with sidewalks. Walk facing oncoming traffic; you want to avoid being followed and surprised from behind by an attacker in a vehicle.
- Always walk down the middle of the sidewalk to reduce the chances of being ambushed by someone hiding in a doorway or between parked cars.
- If you're feeling uneasy, walk in the street rather than on the sidewalk.
- Be aware that portable headphones impair your ability to hear and sense potential dangers.
- If you believe someone is following you on foot, cross the street, turn and walk in the opposite direction, or take refuge in any crowded place (market, restaurant, building lobby). Whenever possible, align yourself with other people.
- If someone in a car is following you, turn and walk or run in the opposite direction, then get to a safe place.

- Don't be predictable; vary your routine. If you walk to work or jog every day, try to vary your timetable and route.

Protect yourself from robbery:

- Never carry large amounts of cash.
- Whenever possible, carry items such as money, credit cards, and housekeys on your person rather than in a purse or wallet. Purses can be snatched; wallets can be lifted by pickpockets.
- Never wear expensive jewelry that may attract the attention of a mugger.
- Carry your purse under your arm and close to your body, or wear a fanny pack.
- Never place the strap of a shoulder bag around your neck. Although this may discourage some purse snatchers, you run the greater risk of being seriously injured if a thief does attempt to grab your bag.
- If a mugger wants your purse, wallet, or jewelry, *give it up.* Never risk your personal safety for money or possessions.

Automated Teller Machines (ATMs):

- Avoid using ATMs whenever possible! ATM users are regular targets of theft and assault. Try to handle your financial business inside the bank.
- If you do use an ATM, exercise caution. Stay alert and aware of your surroundings at all times. Continue to look behind you and around you until you've completed your transaction.
- Whenever possible, have someone with you when you use an ATM.
- Never use an ATM after dark.

Safety in buildings:

- If you see strangers loitering nearby as you approach a secure building (your office or apartment complex, for example), delay your entrance until you feel safe. Many intruders wait for someone to unlock a security door, then force their way inside.

- When you wait for an elevator, stand six to eight feet back from the doors. This will give you a greater margin of safety if an aggressor comes at you from inside the elevator.
- Never enter an elevator if there is a lone, male stranger inside.
- If you're on an elevator and feel uncomfortable at any time, get off at the nearest floor.

In parking lots and garages:

- Exercise caution! Parking lots of all kinds—and especially underground garages—are favored by many attackers.
- Always survey your surroundings *before* walking to your car. If you spot someone suspicious loitering nearby, or if you simply feel uncomfortable, don't leave a store, home, or office until you feel safe. Ask someone in the building to accompany you to your car.
- Have your car key in your hand. Many people are attacked while searching their pockets or digging through their purses.
- *Before* getting inside, always check the front and back seats, and look underneath and around your car. Attackers and carjackers favor these hiding places.
- If you're approached by someone while getting into your car, get in immediately, lock the doors, and lay on the horn to attract attention.
- Avoid walking close to parked cars and vans.
- In selecting a parking space, put safety over convenience. Whenever possible, choose a space that is well-lit and/or close to outside activity, such as a security post.

SAFETY BEHIND THE WHEEL

- Never offer a lift to a stranger, male *or* female.
- Keep your car in good running condition.

- Always be sure you have plenty of fuel to reach your destination. Never let your fuel level drop towards empty.
- Know where you're going! The lost motorist can easily become the stranded motorist. Be sure to carry money, a credit card, and loose change in case you need to use a pay phone.
- If you need to pull over to check a map or get your bearings, do so only in a well-lit place where plenty of other people are around. Avoid stopping at highway rest stops at night.
- If you can afford it, BUY A CELLULAR PHONE. This needn't be an extravagance if you reserve it for emergency use only. A cellular phone has tremendous value in any vehicular emergency. It enables you to summon help if you're ever lost, stranded, threatened, or involved in an accident.

If you have car trouble:

- Pull to the right shoulder of the road. Even if your radiator is spewing steam or your car has one or more flat tires, always try to get to the right shoulder. Never stop in a traffic lane, and especially not in the inside lane.
- If possible, try to stop in a well-lit, well-traveled area. Turn on your emergency lights and raise the hood to attract the attention of police, then remain in your car with the doors locked. DON'T turn on an interior light. If you have a cellular phone, use it to call for assistance.
- If a stranger approaches to offer you assistance, don't get out of your car, and don't ever accept a lift. Instead, ask him or her to drive to the nearest phone and call for help. If you feel uncomfortable or threatened—and don't want to appear helpless—tell the stranger that help is on the way.
- If you've broken down at night or on a rarely traveled road, remaining inside your car may not be the safest thing to do. You might be better off getting out of your car and hiding in a location where you can keep an eye on your car without being seen by others.
- If you think your car may be hit from behind, again, get out and move to a safe area nearby. Be aware that your car

may be rear-ended or sideswiped even when it is parked on the shoulder of a highway or freeway.

- Never leave the vicinity of your car unless you know where you are going. If you spot a freeway call box, open business, or off-ramp and decide to walk to it, remain conscious of your vulnerability. Keep off of the road *and* off of the shoulder to avoid attracting attention.
- If a law enforcement officer approaches your car, ask to see photo identification before unlocking your door. Years ago, one attacker in the San Diego area disguised himself as a police officer, complete with uniform, badge, and marked patrol car.

If you're involved in an accident:

- Be aware that not all accidents are genuine; some sideswipes and fenderbenders are staged as a prelude to armed rape, robbery, and car theft.
- If you feel uncomfortable in the location of the accident, and your car is operable, tell the other motorist to follow you to a safe place. Then notify police.
- If the other driver makes you feel nervous or threatened, forget the dialogue and drive to a safe place. Contact police from there. You may leave the scene of the accident if you believe your personal safety is at risk.

To prevent carjacking:

- If you're followed while in your car, never pull over or drive home. Drive to the nearest police station, fire station, gas station, or open business, then lay on the horn to attract attention.
- If someone bumps you from behind, DO NOT stop, get out of your car, or confront the other driver. This ruse is used by "bumper rapists," by "bump 'n' rob" armed robbers, and (especially) by carjackers.
- Keep car doors locked at all times.
- Keep windows up whenever possible.

- Be aware that carjackers usually work in teams, sometimes with a female partner.

- Be aware that an attacker may use a ruse to persuade you to step out of your car. He may ask to borrow your jumper cables, for example, or warn you that you have a flat or wobbly tire.

- If a stranger approaches your car and you feel comfortable speaking to him or her, crack your window a couple of inches but never roll it down the whole way. At the same time, keep your motor running, and do not get out of your car.

- If a stranger approaches your car and you feel uncomfortable or threatened in any way, *hit the gas*. You're always safer moving than staying still.

- Check your side and rearview mirrors regularly. Carjackers often follow unsuspecting targets home from restaurants, banks, and shopping malls.

- Keep all valuables off seats and out of sight. This includes a purse or briefcase.

- Be advised that while expensive, high-profile cars often attract the attention of car thieves, they are not the only targets.

- Remember that the quickest route is not always the safest one. Avoid driving in areas that are unfamiliar to you, or seldom traveled. Avoid high-crime areas; be aware that graffiti on walls and buildings is often a sign of local gang activity.

- Keep your car keys on a separate ring from your house keys. The person who steals your car may later try to rob your house.

- Keep your car registration *hidden* in your car. An auto registration left in the glove compartment is easily found and provides too much information to a thief.

- Exercise caution at stoplights; whenever possible, try to leave some space between your car and the one ahead of you. Many carjackings are initiated when the victim's car is "boxed in" by other traffic.

- If an armed assailant wants your car, *let him take it*. Hand over your keys (do not throw them), then get to safety ASAP.

If you're confronted while seated behind the wheel, exit the car through the passenger door (if possible), then get to safety. Immediately notify police.

SAFETY AT THE OFFICE

- Whenever possible, avoid staying alone at your office after hours. If you must work late, move to an area where you can see and hear others, and notify security personnel that you are in the building.
- If you must leave your workplace after hours or after dark, ask a colleague or security guard to walk you to your car.
- Familiarize yourself with the security regulations and policies of your company. (Does your company screen visitors to the building? Is there someone on site after normal business hours?) If you have any safety concerns, report them to your employer. Management has a legal responsibility to provide for a safe and secure workplace.
- If you spot someone in your workplace during business hours whom you do not recognize, or whose behavior seems at all suspicious, don't be reluctant to confront him or her (*"Can I help you?"*). All too often, an attacker will "cruise" an office building looking for potential victims.
- Familiarize yourself with all exits in your building and especially on your floor, including doorways, windows, stairwells, and public and service elevators.
- Have a definite plan in the event of an emergency.
- If you are verbally or physically threatened by a co-worker at any time, notify management, human resources, and security personnel immediately.

SAFETY WHILE TRAVELING

- Travel with others whenever possible.
- Never flash cash or jewelry in public.
- Never use your home address or phone number on luggage tags; whenever possible, use business information instead. Be assured that if your luggage is lost and later found, it

will not be "automatically" sent to the address you have supplied; that address will be used for identification purposes only.

- Familiarize yourself with all hotel exits: from your room, your floor, and from the building itself.
- Use a travel door lock (available at many locksmiths and hardware stores) when staying in hotel rooms. Many hotel rooms are dangerously easy to break into.

Hands-On Courses and Training

It's not unusual for women to ask my advice in selecting a hands-on self-defense course. There are so many different programs to choose from, selecting the best one for you can be truly confusing.

The key words here are "best for you," because the right program will not necessarily be the most expensive or the most popular, or even have the most experienced instructor. It will be the course that best fits your special needs. So when people ask my advice about choosing a program, the first thing I ask them is, "What are you interested in? What are you looking for? What do you hope to get out of the program?"

Generally speaking, if you want to learn basic self-defense, take a self-defense course. While many martial arts provide excellent conditioning, flexibility, discipline, and spiritual benefits, not all are designed to train you in real-life street survival.

At the same time, shy away from programs that teach *only* physical self-defense. As you've learned from reading this book, physical techniques are only one small part of personal empowerment. It's just as important—if not more so—to learn all the nonphysical forms of personal protection, such as boundary-setting, assertiveness, de-escalation, and preventive safety measures, just to name a few.

Selecting an Assault Prevention Program

If you want to pursue an assault prevention program that provides street survival skills similar to those I've provided throughout this book, call your local police department or rape crisis center for a referral. Many police departments and support agencies are familiar with the training programs in their area.

Once you get a referral, contact the instructor or group to find out everything you can about the program. If you like what you hear, ask to sit in on a class. If they won't allow you to sit in free of charge, take that as a negative. Whenever possible, meet the person who would be teaching your class. You should feel completely comfortable with the instructor, especially if it's a hands-on program where he or she will be touching you in unfamiliar ways. Trust your intuition: if you feel uncomfortable about either the instructor or the program, go somewhere else.

Whether you get your information over the phone or in person, here are the kinds of questions you want answered:

Who facilitates the program? The instructor is absolutely crucial to the success of any program, so find out about his or her education, experience, and training. Ask for references, and check those references out. Whenever possible, speak to people the instructor has trained. There's no substitute for strong personal recommendations.

Try to learn about the instructor's background; this is likely to influence the program itself. For example, if he or she is a former police officer, the program might have a strong crime-prevention slant; on the other hand, if the instructor is or was a rape crisis counselor, the program might focus on rape to the exclusion of other forms of assault. Finally, make sure that the instructor you meet will be your instructor throughout the program. Some programs have three or four instructors and rotate them accordingly, so you may end up with one instructor one week, and a different instructor the next. In my opinion, this is not an ideal situation. If at all possible, find a course where you have the same instructor from beginning to end.

What is the primary focus of the program: assault prevention or martial arts? Nearly every martial arts instructor I've met thinks that he's an expert on assault prevention for women, but that doesn't always mean that he is. There's a skill to teaching assault prevention with expertise and sensitivity, and it differs greatly from teaching any kind of martial art. Therefore, try to find someone whose experience extends beyond martial arts training. For example, I have a background not only in Kung Fu San Soo and the art of street fighting, but in public health education and women's self-defense.

I've had the opportunity to sit in on many different types of self-defense programs, and while there are many caring, highly qualified instructors out there, I've also met my share of incompetents. In my experience, these people tend towards one of two extremes: either macho, insensitive men who are law enforcement or martial arts professionals, or militant feminists who see men as the "enemy" and believe that only women can teach women's self-defense. Instructors with extreme attitudes or rigid political agendas tend to be the worst kind of instructors, so try to avoid them.

How long has the program been in existence? In other words, would you be one of their first students, or have they "graduated" many students before you? Be warned: just because a program has been around for years doesn't necessarily mean that it's good. Whether it's been operating for one year or ten, the important thing is that it's been around long enough to acquire a good local reputation and positive word of mouth.

How many people have they trained, and what percentage of those were women? Just because a program offers assault prevention training to women doesn't mean that the program is *tailored* for women.

I make no apologies for my opinion that women should attend a class designed with them in mind. This is not sexist, but realistic. When it comes to self-defense training, men and women have different needs. In my experience, women have an apprehension of being assaulted which men simply do not have, and you need an instructor who is cognizant of those fears and sensitive to them. Also, men are generally taller, bigger, and have more upper-body strength than women, so women should learn to defend themselves in ways that not only overcome those male "advantages," but make them irrelevant.

Don't attend a course that mixes male and female students. In my experience, this creates tension in the class that would not otherwise exist. For example, I've found that women are significantly less comfortable doing role-playing exercises when men are present. Meanwhile, the presence of female students tends to bring out the domineering side of many men.

At the same time, avoid any class where the instructor seems to believe that women are weaker than men or less capable of defending themselves. The first thing I tell my female students is, "You can do this. You can fight." If you don't get this message from your instructor, find a different instructor.

How long is the course? Self-defense and empowerment programs come in all shapes and sizes. You can sign up for an intensive one-day course, for example, or a once-a-week course spread out over six or eight weeks. The question you really need to ask yourself is, "How much time can I realistically devote to the process?" Completion is the key when it comes to any program. I'd rather see you complete a one-day class than sign up for an eight-week course and drop out after the third week.

If one day is all you can spare, that's fine. Don't let anyone tell you that one-day courses are a waste of time or are too short to be of any value. The great majority of my own programs are one-day. I spend a very intensive eight hours with six or seven women, with practically no distractions or interruptions. And believe me, those students learn a great deal. The intensity of a one-day course has certain advantages. Whenever I offer once-a-week classes spread out over several weeks, I inevitably lose some students in the process. Learning personal empowerment can be an anxiety-producing process, and it can be hard to sustain a commitment over a six- or eight-week period.

How much does the course cost? Just because a course is expensive is no guarantee that it's good. What's more, if it's being taught in a plush studio, a sizeable chunk of your tuition may be going towards paying the rent. Prices vary: some YWCA chapters offer programs for between $20 and $30, while some courses lasting several weeks can run from $400 to $500. Price is a factor for most of us, but quality should take precedence. Instead of bargain-hunting, I'd rather see you find the best course for you and then go from there.

How many people are in a class? If the program is hands-on, your class should have no more than 10 people in it. I don't care if the lead instructor has one assistant with him or three, if there are more than 10 people in the class, you're just not going to get the individualized attention that you need. On the other hand, if the program is not hands-on, the number of students is irrelevant.

Does the course include hands-on training? There's nothing like getting some hands-on experience, period. Learning the theory of various techniques is never a waste of time, but getting the chance to practice them on a real human being simply can't be beat.

There's also no substitute for having a man in the class with whom the students can practice their role-playing exercises and physical techniques. Whether he is the primary instructor or just an assistant, it always helps to practice on the "real thing."

What kind of techniques are taught? Be sure that the program offers its students the opportunity to do role-playing exercises in physical *and* verbal skills. For a program to be thorough, it must include practice in all types of empowerment and protective techniques. Meanwhile, the physical techniques should be *street-oriented*. If the program focuses on kicks and punches, but not street-fighting techniques like vital-target attacks to the eye or throat, then you won't be getting the training you need.

In recent years, we've seen the emergence of classes for women that combine aerobic workouts with training in boxing or the martial arts. Some examples are "Boxersize" (a combination of boxing and fitness exercises) and "Karobics" (combining karate and aerobics). If you're drawn to these kinds of programs because you want to get a good aerobic workout, fine. Don't suppose for a minute, however, that they will teach you street-survival skills, because they won't.

Although parts of the process may make you anxious, especially if you have previously suffered an assault, learning how to protect yourself should be a positive, uplifting experience overall. You should find it enjoyable, educational and challenging, and you should feel safe and encouraged in the teaching environment. Just because you're learning how to protect yourself doesn't mean that the learning process itself has to be a dark, depressing, frightening experience. You want a program that is going to empower you not just physically but emotionally, spiritually, and psychologically. Its benefits should not begin and end with personal protection but should cross over into other aspects of your life. If you enroll in a program and find it doesn't meet these criteria, don't be reluctant to drop out and find another program that does.

Fighting Techniques: A Capsule Summary

It's perhaps inevitable that in the months and years to come, you will start to forget some of the things about self-defense that you have learned from this book. Fortunately, there are a few things you can do that will help to keep you current.

First, try to practice your self-defense techniques with a partner. There's nothing like getting some hands-on experience, and guidelines for practicing safely and effectively can be found later in this chapter.

Second, periodically read through the capsule summary that follows. Look upon it as a 10-minute refresher course that will help to keep you prepared. One word of caution: this summary is intended only as a "companion guide" to supplement the more detailed explanations I provided earlier; it is *not* intended as a substitute. Therefore, do *not* share this summary with someone else until they have a full understanding of each principle and technique.

ESSENTIAL PRINCIPLES FOR SELF-DEFENSE

- Fight with 100 percent commitment
- Fight for your survival
- Fight "smart"
- Cause pain
- Get to safety as soon as possible

RULES OF ENGAGEMENT

- Stay close
- Grab and hold on
- "Set" your weight
- Keep breathing
- Be patient

YOUR NATURAL WEAPONS

- Hands (to grab and tear, rather than to punch)
- Elbows
- Knees
- Feet
- Head
- Teeth

AN ATTACKER'S REACTIONS TO PAIN

- His hands will move *towards* his pain
- His body will recoil *away* from pain
- He may scream

THE "BLINDSIDE" TECHNIQUE

Essential for any surprise attack to the throat or head area ("What he cannot see, he cannot stop")

- Get close
- Bring your attacking hand up the front or side of your attacker's body until you reach your target

ATTENTION-GETTERS

Bites. Aim to cause not just pain, but damage. Bites to any part of the body will cause pain, but especially vulnerable targets include the lips, cheeks, inside of the upper arm, chest area, throat, inner thigh, penis, and testicles.

Pinches. Pinch or twist the skin (especially of the inner thigh, or the underside of the upper arm).

Hammer strikes. Make a fist and use the padded part of that fist to strike at the nose, eye, or throat.

Head butts. Slam your attacker's nose with the back of your skull (if he's behind you) or the very top of your forehead (if he's facing you).

Knees. (Depending on your target, either the kneecap, or the portion of your thigh that is *just above* the knee.) Strike the inner or outer thigh, face, ribs, or testicles.

Finger breaks. Grab and bend the finger *back* full force until you hear and feel the break. Note: the small "pinky" finger is the easiest to break.

Kicks. Kick any part of your attacker's leg *below* the knee: ankle, shin, calf, or Achilles' tendon. Always use the ball of your foot (never the toes, unless you're wearing sturdy footwear).

Heel-stomps. Drive your heel down onto your attacker's foot or toes.

Eye pokes. Make a "Boy Scout oath" with your first and second fingers pointing outward, then jab those two fingers into the eye.

Eye-scrapes. Starting from the corner nearest the nose, use your thumb to scrape outward across the eye.

Ear box. Strike the ear with the *palm* of your flattened hand, or strike both ears simultaneously.

Ear tear. Attack one or both ears. Grab the whole ear, dig your fingers into the skin behind it, then rip down towards your hip. *(When attacking the eye or ear, always bring your hand up your attacker's blind side.)*

Groin attacks. Drive a solid knee up between the legs to strike the testicles. Slap the testicles with your hand. Use your fist to hammer-strike the bladder or groin.

VITAL-TARGET ATTACKS

To the EYE

Your action and non-action hands work simultaneously:

- Cup the back of your attacker's neck with your **non-action** hand (right or left), keep your elbows in, and use all your body weight to pull him *down* towards the shoulder of your non-action hand.
- Open your **attacking** hand (in "toast"-like fashion). Drive your thumb into the inside corner of his eye as your fingers grip and squeeze the side of his head.
  Maintain the pressure for five to ten seconds. If your attacker begins to collapse or sag against you, don't try to hold him up: turn his head towards your non-action hand and shove him forcefully to the ground.

To the THROAT (i.e. the windpipe)

- *CAUTION: Attacks to the throat inhibit your attacker's ability to breathe and can actually result in death.*
- *With any attack to the throat, always move your hand up your attacker's blind side.*

THE STRIKE: With fingers curved in a "toast"-like fashion, slam your open hand into the front of the throat. Hit *through* the target.

THE GRAB: Dig your fingers and thumb *into* the windpipe, squeeze with all your strength, and rip outward.

(The strike and grab are most effective when your non-action hand is cupping the back of your attacker's neck and pulling him towards you.)

THE BITE: Wrap both your hands behind your attacker's neck, pull him towards you, and sink your teeth into his windpipe.

To the GROIN:

- *Aim for the testicles, rather than the penis.*
- *Never attempt to KICK a man in the testicles.*
- *With any groin attack, your attacker will double forward at the waist. To avoid knocking heads, stand slightly to his left or right.*
- **STRIKE** the testicles with the palm-heel part of your open hand, with your fingers pointed down.
- If your attacker is wearing loose-fitting pants, **GRAB** the testicles and crush them in your fist. (If he isn't wearing pants, grab and crush the testicles then *tear outward.*)
- With the strike and grab, place your non-action hand on your attacker's lower back or buttocks to give you more leverage and control.
- To **KNEE** the testicles, grab hold of your attacker and drive your knee up *forcefully* between his thighs.

If you are forced to your knees to perform oral copulation—and there's no weapon in evidence—**BITE** deep into his penis, and/or crush his testicles in your fist as you tear outward.

DEFENSES AGAINST SLAPS AND PUNCHES

- *Protecting your head is crucial*
- *Position yourself: get well out of striking distance, or get CLOSE*
- *Always keep your eyes on your attacker; never duck your head, close your eyes, or look away*

To protect your head:

- Wrap your arms around him in a bear hug and tuck your head into his chest (until you're ready to counterattack)
  Or:
- Cup the back of your neck with both hands, press your forearms flush against your ears, and point your elbows towards your attacker
  Or:

- (best idea) GO ON THE OFFENSIVE.

ESCAPING GRABS, HOLDS & CHOKES

Don't:

- try to pull away
- fight your attacker's strength

Do:

- take a deep breath
- set your weight
- get close
- CAUSE PAIN

GRABS

If an attacker grabs your arm:

- twist your arm up and around in a circular motion
- (best of all) use your free hand or another natural weapon to CAUSE PAIN

If he grabs your wrist:

- close your captured hand into a fist, grab that fist with your free hand, then pull back towards your shoulder
- (best of all) use your free hand or another natural weapon to CAUSE PAIN

If he grabs your hair:

- don't reach for it or try to pull away
- do move in the direction you're being pulled (stay with him)
- get as close as you can, then CAUSE PAIN

HOLDS FROM THE REAR

If your arms are *pinned:*

- heel-stomp down onto his toes or instep
- scrape your heel down his shin
- drive an elbow into his ribs or solar plexus
- slam your head back against his nose
- reach back to pinch or twist the skin of his groin or inner thigh
- reach back to grab and crush his testicles

If your arms are *free,* you can also:

- pinch or twist the skin of his forearms or hands
- grab and break his pinky finger

HOLDS FROM THE FRONT ("BEAR HUGS")

If your arms are *free:*

- tear an ear
- use your teeth
- strike or grab his throat
- drive your thumb into his eye

If your arms are *pinned:*

- knee your attacker between the legs
- grab his groin
- head-butt his nose
- bite into his shoulder, neck, cheek, lip, tongue (whatever you can get to)

CHOKES

- *Fight back IMMEDIATELY*
- *Don't try to pull his hands or arm away: CAUSE PAIN*

If you're choked at arm's length (and need to bring your attacker closer):

- pinch or twist the skin and hair under his bicep or underarm
- place your hands on top of the crook of his elbow and pull down and towards you

If you're choked from behind:

- reach back to pinch, twist, grab or strike his groin
- stomp down on his instep
- scrape your heel against his shin, or heel-kick back into his shin

If his arm is wrapped around your throat:

- grab hold of his arm and hang on it, using all your body weight to bring it down and towards your chest
  then:
- CAUSE PAIN

If your arms are *free*, you can also:

- pinch or twist the skin of his forearms or hands
- grab his pinky finger and break it
- *If you can't use your arms or hands, use your legs or head: take advantage of what's available.*

MAKING "DISADVANTAGES" WORK FOR YOU

If you're **backed against a wall,** it means you:

- have added support behind you
- can use the wall as a weapon
- cannot be attacked from behind

If you're **"cornered,"** it means you:

- have *two* walls for support
- have *two* walls to use as weapons
- cannot be attacked from the back or the side

If you are **seated:**

- fight from that position
- zero in on accessible targets (e.g. the groin)
- use your chair as a secondary weapon

If you're **on the ground,** it means:

- you have support beneath you
- you can't be injured by falling, tripping, or being shoved off your feet

If you end up on the ground, *fight from that position*. Don't try to get up or push your attacker off you.

If you are **pinned down** at the wrists or arms (and want to get one or both arms free):

- yell at the top of your lungs
- bite into his hand, wrist, or forearm
- bite into his lip (if he's trying to kiss you)
- shoot your arms above your head (keeping them on the ground *at all times)*
- simultaneously straighten one arm *up* (towards your head) and one arm *down* (towards your feet), keeping both arms on the ground
     or:
- WAIT for him to release your arm(s)

As soon as you have **one arm free:**

- hook the back of your attacker's neck to control his body and free your other arm, then attack the EYE

MULTIPLE ATTACKERS

- go on the offensive
- go after them one at a time
- go after the attacker closest to you
- immediately cause serious pain and damage

then:

- use Attacker #1 as a shield against Attacker #2
- once Attacker #1 is "finished," go after Attacker #2

Whenever possible, back up against a wall or solid structure.

ATTACKERS WITH WEAPONS

- *Exercise caution with any armed attacker; resist only in life-or-death situations.*
- *If he wants your money or car, don't resist.*
- *If he drops his weapon or lays it aside, don't go after it! Focus on the man, not the weapon.*

If you choose to fight someone who has a **gun:**

- get very close
- make nonthreatening contact with the weapon hand
  (then do three things simultaneously:)
- grab on to his wrist
- deflect the weapon hand in one direction and move your body in another
- cause SERIOUS pain (grab his windpipe, scrape his eye, or knee him in the testicles)

Depending on visibility (daylight versus darkness) and your distance from your attacker, you can also run from someone who has a gun.

If you choose to fight someone who has a **knife:**

- make nonthreatening contact with the knife hand *(then do three things simultaneously:)*
- tightly grip his wrist
- move the weapon hand away from your body (if he's in front of you) or hold it close against your body (if he's in back with the knife to your throat)
- use your other hand to CAUSE PAIN
- *Remember that you can be stabbed inadvertently by a knife.*
- *Exercise extreme caution if the knife is near your throat.*
- *Be ready to risk minor pain and injury to avoid major injury and death.*

Practicing With a Partner

You can practice your self-defense techniques with a man or with a woman. You may also want to experiment with partners of varying height, weight, and build.

Note: The only reason you practice is to develop a feel for the balance, leverage, and movement that each technique requires. You are not practicing these techniques to see if they "work," because they will *only* work if you inflict pain.

Here's how to practice safely and effectively:

1. Have your partner face you, with his hands at his sides. (For simplicity's sake, we'll assume that your partner is a man.) Reassure your partner that he will not be hurt by any of your techniques.
2. Execute each step of each technique in SLOW MOTION.
3. Don't physically connect with your target. For example, if you want to practice a knee to the groin, slowly grab hold of your partner's shirt, slowly bring your leg up between his legs, then stop an inch short of actual physical contact.
4. If you would like to experience the full power and range of motion of two particular techniques—the knee to the groin, and the open-hand strike to the throat—just "adjust" your target. For example, bring your knee up along the

outside of your partner's leg, or aim your hand-strike at the "airspace" next to his neck.

5. As you practice each technique, your partner should simply stand there. At no time should he try to "test" you, or otherwise resist.

6. If you want to practice escaping a grab or hold, ask your partner to restrain you *gently*. No force or pressure should be applied.

If you don't have a partner to practice with, you can use an imaginary figure. Practice taking a few deep breaths, setting your weight, and using a blindside technique to reach "his" head. Practice cupping the back of his neck with one hand as you attack his eye with the other. You'll have the technique down in no time. And remember: with an imaginary partner, you can practice at full-speed, and with maximum power.

RESOURCES

National Organization for Victim Assistance (NOVA)
1-800-TRY-NOVA
(1-800-879-6682)

This 24-hour hotline provides free crisis counseling to victims of violent crime* throughout the United States and Canada. It also provides referrals for attorneys, therapists, counselors, and other victim-related support services in your local area. (Spanish-speaking advocates available.)

Victims of domestic violence are asked to call the number below.

National Domestic Violence Hotline
1-800-799-SAFE
(1-800-799-7233)

A 24-hour hotline that provides referrals on shelters and domestic violence programs available throughout the United States, Puerto Rico, and Canada. English and Spanish-speaking advocates are available, along with access to over 140 other foreign language advocates.

Hearing-impaired individuals are asked to call 1-800-787-3224.

RECOMMENDED READING

DEFENDING OURSELVES: A Guide to Prevention, Self-Defense, and Recovery From Rape by Rosalind Wiseman. (New York: Noonday Press, 1991.) As the title implies, this eloquently written book focuses primarily on rape. Particularly valuable are those sections that discuss the mental and emotional recovery process and how to deal with police, hospitals, and the courts in the aftermath of rape.

HER WITS ABOUT HER: Self-Defense Success Stories by Women edited by Denise Caignon and Gail Groves. (New York: Harper & Row, 1987.) An absolutely inspiring book in which real women describe how they defended themselves with techniques ranging from the ordinary to the spectacular. A real antidote to the myth of the helpless female.

THE VERBALLY ABUSIVE RELATIONSHIP: How to Recognize It and How to Respond by Patricia Evans. (Holbrook, MA: Bob Adams Inc., 1992.) Hands down, the best book I've read on identifying and stopping the many forms of verbal abuse.

STRONG ON DEFENSE: Survival Rules to Protect You and

Your Family From Crime by Sanford Strong. (New York: Pocket Books, 1996.) A 20-year police veteran, the author's specialty was training fellow officers in defense and survival skills. While he focuses on the very worst-case scenarios of violent crime, this is a very readable, no-holds-barred look at the face of crime today. Of particular value are the true case histories which illustrate what to do and what not to do in a variety of situations.

HOW TO PROTECT YOURSELF FROM CRIME by Ira A. Lipman. (Chicago: Contemporary Books, 1989.) Written by a leader in the security industry, this book covers just about every safety measure you can take to protect you and your family from crime.

MINDHUNTER: Inside the FBI's Elite Serial Crime Unit and *JOURNEY INTO DARKNESS,* both by John Douglas and Mark Olshaker. (New York: Scribner, 1995 and 1997 respectively.) Co-author Douglas was the FBI special agent who pioneered criminal profiling, and both of these books provide a fascinating look into the psychology and methods of serial rapists, child molesters, and murderers.

For any woman who has been the victim of domestic violence, or who simply wants to know more about the subject, I recommend any of the following: *THE BATTERED WOMAN* by Lenore E. Walker (New York: Harper & Row, 1979), *THE BATTERED WOMAN'S SURVIVAL GUIDE: Breaking the Cycle* by Jan Berliner Statman (Dallas, TX: Taylor Publishing, 1995), and *DEFENDING OUR LIVES: Getting Away From Domestic Violence & Staying Safe* by Susan Murphy-Milano (New York: Anchor Books/Doubleday, 1996). Of specific interest to teenagers is *IN LOVE AND IN DANGER: A Teen's Guide to Breaking Free of Abusive Relationships* by Barrie Levy (Seattle, WA: Seal Press, 1993).

STALKED: Breaking the Silence on the Crime of Stalking in America by Melita Schaum and Karen Parrish. (New York: Pocket Books, 1995.) The first book I've found that deals exclusively with this issue. Thorough and highly informative.

SOFTPOWER!: How to Speak up, Set Limits, and Say No Without Losing Your Lover, Your Job, Or Your Friends by Maria Arapakis. (New York: Warner Books Inc., 1990.) An assertiveness guide to help you handle everyday challenges. Continuing along the same personal empowerment theme is ***WOMEN'S SELF-ESTEEM: Understanding and Improving the Way We Think and Feel About Ourselves*** by Linda Tschirhart Sanford and Mary Ellen Donovan (New York: Penguin Books, 1985.).

BODY LANGUAGE by Julius Fast. (New York: Pocket Books, 1971.) More than 25 years and three million copies later, the author's observations on the "silent communication" of body language still make for informative and entertaining reading.

ZEN IN THE MARTIAL ARTS by Joe Hyams. (New York: Bantam, 1982.) Don't let the title mislead you; this is no "how-to" manual. Rather, the author uses the martial arts as a metaphor for how to live your life and attain your full potential. A quick and spiritually uplifting read.

A Note From the Author

Thousands of women have benefited from my lectures, seminars, and workshops. If you would like to bring my program to your company, organization, or community, or would like more information on my services and products, please write or call:

Al Marrewa
1015 Gayley Avenue, Suite 191
Los Angeles, California 90024

1-800-806-4986 or 310-358-3612